Failing Government
Taketh Away

Jerry L. Rhoads

Copyright © 2015 by Jerry L. Rhoads.

Library of Congress Control Number: 2014920005
ISBN: Hardcover   978-1-5035-1336-5
              Softcover   978-1-5035-1337-2
              eBook   978-1-5035-1338-9

All rights reserved. No part of this book may be reproduced or transmitted in any form or by any means, electronic or mechanical, including photocopying, recording, or by any information storage and retrieval system, without permission in writing from the copyright owner.

Any people depicted in stock imagery provided by Thinkstock are models, and such images are being used for illustrative purposes only.
Certain stock imagery © Thinkstock.

Print information available on the last page.

Rev. date: 06/09/2015

To order additional copies of this book, contact:
Xlibris
1-888-795-4274
www.Xlibris.com
Orders@Xlibris.com
661197

Contents

FOREWORD 5
PREFACE 9
MONOPSONY GRAPH 12
ACKNOWLEDGMENTS 13

PART I—AMERICA THE DUTIFUL

DUTY NO. 1—MONOPSONY GAME RULES AND REGS 17
DUTY NO. 2—WHO IS THE BIGGEST BULLY (in China's Shop)? 36
DUTY NO. 3—BIGGEST BULLY FAILURE 52

PART II—CATCH 23

CHAPTER ONE: MONOPSONY DISREGARDS THE RULE
        OF LAW 70
CHAPTER TWO: WILL MONOPSONY CARE FIX
        HEALTH-CARE PROBLEMS? 83
CHAPTER THREE: HOW GOVERNMENT AND
        POLITICIANS MONOPSONIZE AND
        BRUTALIZE SMALL BUSINESSES 95
CHAPTER FOUR: ENTERPRISE'S FIRST MOVE: LINK
        INCOME TO OUTCOME 108
CHAPTER FIVE: HOW ENTERPRISE HEALTH CARE
        WINS THE MONOPSONY GAME 115
CHAPTER SIX: HOW GOVERNMENT MONOPSONY
        HEALTH CARE SINS 122
CHAPTER SEVEN: HOW ENTERPRISE HEALTH CARE LOSES 134
CHAPTER EIGHT: HOW OUTPUT-BASED HEALTH CARE
        WINS 159
CHAPTER NINE: MONOPSONY COMMITS FRAUD AND
        ABUSE 163
CHAPTER TEN: ENTERPRISE HEALTH CARE PASSES GO 177

PART III—"GOTCHA"

CHAPTER ELEVEN: "GOTCHA RULES THE SHOP" 183
CHAPTER TWELVE: "GOTCHA" REGULATIONS
    MONOPSONY WINS AGAIN.. 193
CHAPTER THIRTEEN: ALL-AMERICAN RESTORATIVE CARE.... 202
CHAPTER FOURTEEN: BIGGEST BULLY TRICK:
    THE DEATH OF ENTERPRISE 207
CHAPTER FIFTEEN: PUNISHMENT FOR LOSING
    MONOPSONY GAME 214
CHAPTER SIXTEEN: HOW TO STOP THE BULLY........................ 222
CHAPTER SEVENTEEN: BIGGEST BULLY IN IOWA..................... 225
CHAPTER EIGHTEEN: HOW TO WIN THE MONOPSONY
    GAME AND DEFEAT THE BIGGEST BULLY 229

THE LAST CHAPTER 246
AFTERWORD 249
EXHIBIT A—The Real Victims of the Monopsony........................ 253
SUMMARY 261
INDEX 265

FOREWORD

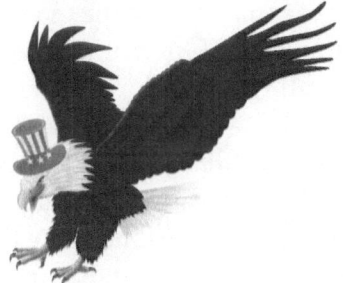

FAILING GOVERNMENT TAKETH AWAY

On the cover Uncle Sam, personified by the eagle from the dollar bill, as Big Bully Government Taketh Away, when it sees a threat or disagreement. This is a story of the Rhoads family victimized, defamed and financially punished by big government for minor infractions by taking away their constitutional right to due process of law. The author has coined this as Catch 23.

There are many health care providers being bullied and victimized by our failing government, taking away freedoms of enterprising Americans', small businesses, patients, families, employees and communities because of enforcement of health care services rules and regulations and not adhering to the Rule of Law and Administrative Procedures Act. It mandates the conduct of the regulators must not be arbitrary and capricious. The proof of them violating these principles are detailed in the case of the Rhoads owned skilled nursing facilities versus the State of Iowa, the State of Arkansas and the Federal Department of Health and Human Services as detailed in Chapters 16 and 17 on behalf of the victims described in pages 257 through 262.

>Victim #1 All-American Care of Little Rock
>Victim #2 All-American Care of Muscatine
>Victim #3 All-American Care of Washington

Interview of author:

Why this book and why now? Well the people that seem to make a difference are victims of some catastrophe or violent disservice. Since I see my family victimized by Government regulators, it is time to speak up, stand up or fall for everything forward.

Is there really a Monopsony Game ... is it really a word? Look it up in Webster, it is a market form in which only one buyer interfaces with many sellers. I did develop a Monopsony Board game. It shows how the buyer of last resort regulates and intimidates the provider of the care into submission.

Is this why you liken Government to being the biggest Bully here and abroad? You can arrive at your own conclusions as you also fall victim to 40,000 laws being passed by the lawmakers each year reducing the freedoms of enterprising individuals and businesses.

What is the solution? Downsize government by privatizing agencies that inhibit Enterprise and prevent innovation and creativity. Then the private agencies can collaborate not suffocate technology.

Where do we start? Read my lips it's Health Care services.

Why do you pick health care first rather than the post office? Because it is the second largest agency in the Federal Government behind the Department of Defense.

The health-care industry is vast. It is costly and grossly inefficient. How could I make such an audacious statement? Having been in and around the health-care business for fifty-two years, I feel that I have some insight into the reasons for the current state of affairs.

Conglomerates, under the auspices of Obama Care, are taking over the majority of the providers. Large insurance companies are going to be the emerging ACOs, an acronym for accountable care organizations. The federal and state governments are at the end of their wits and budget means, all because the health of the country is considered an inalienable right while, at the same time, it is big business.

While America is number ONE in cost per capita and thirty-eighth in quality, statistically, Americans spend more money on their health care than anything else but food. But the consumption of the health-care dollar is predominately not paid for by the consumer. The middlemen, so to speak, make the forces of free enterprise moot. Consumers are bystanders in the relationship between purchase and quality because they do not directly pay for the product.

This phenomenon is called monopsony. The consumer is not the buyer. But the buyer is almost singly dominant. This is the reverse of monopoly, where the seller has the last say. This is not Microsoft at work. It is the federal and state Medicare and Medicaid programs that buy upward of seventy five percent of all health-care service products. Under the Obama nation, government will be the purchaser of last resort for all Americans.

Ingeniously, the insurance industry convinced the federal government in 1966 that the only fair and equitable manner to fund and pay for health care for the elderly and disabled was to pay reimbursable costs including a markup for overhead and return on equity. Most of the providers, in those days, were not-for-profit hospitals and sole-practitioner doctors. This method lasted until 1989, when it was changed, in terms of payment, for hospital care and the emerging continuum of services for the elderly population.

DRGs (diagnosis-related groupings) set a price for a diagnostic group without regard to what it costs the hospital. This political maneuver has turned the tables on the providers and forced them to look at cost and economize. The same method is now being embraced for all facets of health care: DRGs for inpatient care, OPUs for outpatient care, RUGs for long-term care, RVUs for physician care, RUGs for nursing-home care, and RIUs for rehabilitative care.

This should have converted the entire health-care industry from a cost-plus economic equation to a managed competition where providers are **pitted against government-fixed prices. Unfortunately, all of health care doesn't have to analyze and cost each service product and be accountable for their cost effectiveness and managerial efficiency. Instead they get paid for esoteric input units not output units depicting outcomes or positive results.**

In order to work, it requires standardization of terms, product-type definitions for cost controls, and activity-based cost accounting systems to value the product costs and manage the margins against the fixed prices. Then enterprise has to learn how to win the monopsony game in spite of the biggest bully in the game—Uncle Sam and his fifty governors.

PREFACE

The following is quoted from a newspaper article published in the Orlando Sentinel, *"545 vs. 300,000,000 People" by Charley Reese.*

- Politicians are the only people in the world who create problems and then campaign against them.
- Have you ever wondered, if both the Democrats and the Republicans are against deficits, WHY do we have deficits?
- Have you ever wondered, if all the politicians are against inflation and high taxes, WHY do we have inflation and high taxes?
- You and I don't propose a federal budget. The President does.
- You and I don't have the Constitutional authority to vote on appropriations. The House of Representatives does.
- You and I don't write the tax code, Congress does.
- You and I don't set fiscal policy, Congress does.
- You and I don't control monetary policy, the Federal Reserve Bank does.
- Gang of 545 = 100 senators, 435 congressmen, one President, and 9 Supreme Court justices . . . equates to 545 human beings out of 300 million who are directly, legally, morally, and individually responsible for the domestic problems that plague this country." *Why then would we believe that they can solve them?*

I call this the business model of the Board of Directors of the Monopsony!

Monopsony Encourages Consolidation of the Providers

Vertical integration of the long term care providers occurs as the Monopsony empowers the regulators to be tougher on enforcement. Rather than horizontal integration that decentralizes delivery systems and makes enforcement less effective and reinforcement more doable and productive.

Of course I am recommending the complete rejection of the consolidation (pyramid) approach, where America's nursing homes are consolidated into giant centralized conglomerates run by absentee executives who decide to cut costs and services because it is their responsibility to comply with Obama Monopsony Care.

Not only is this approach passé in terms of social structures and government, it is ironically self-destructive to the human element in any business. Though I am not suggesting that we bring back the days of family-run homes, I am suggesting that corporate takeovers for the purpose of being large enough to fend off the power of the Monopsony Game only results in warehousing our elderly. We experienced this in the 1980s when managed care was the name of the game.

Rise and Fall of Consolidation: The resurgence of the Pyramid Age

"We need to get rid of the mom and pops . . . . They are inefficient and poorly run small businesses, and we can build on economies of scale and knowledge of how to succeed in business without even trying." Such was the strategy of the captains of the real estate business who began tearing into nursing homes in the 1980s and overnight built giant conglomerates that I call pyramids. These pyramids cost America its personal patient centered care and hollowed out the very core of quality for the elderly.

It all started with a small-time owner of three nursing homes in California that grew into Beverly Enterprises, which once owned 1,200 nursing homes across the nation and has since imploded due to substandard care and violation of the minimum standards of quality. This paved the way for the classic strategy of acquiring real estate with a business attached—in this case, servicing the growing needs of an aging society. Other operators followed, including Manor Care, Sun Health, Mariner, Kinder Care, National Health, Vencor, Hillhaven, Genesis, and Integrated Health Services. Now it is Avi and Kindred.

Currently, 50 percent of the nursing home industry is owned by chain operators having 20 or more homes. Another 25 percent is owned by religious-based groups who own three or more (Good Samaritan, for example, at one time owned over 200). What that means is that 75 percent of nursing homes have absentee ownership.

What is absentee ownership? It is the organizational structure in which the money decisions are made off-site. The on-site administrator has all the responsibility, limited authority on operational policies, and no authority on money issues.

With the emergence of Obama Care giving rise to more enforcement and money driven care consolidation is inevitable as enterprise fights the dominance of the Monopsony. It didn't work in the 1980s and is destined to fail again. If allowed to evolve it will destroy competition as does Monopoly.

MONOPSONY GRAPH

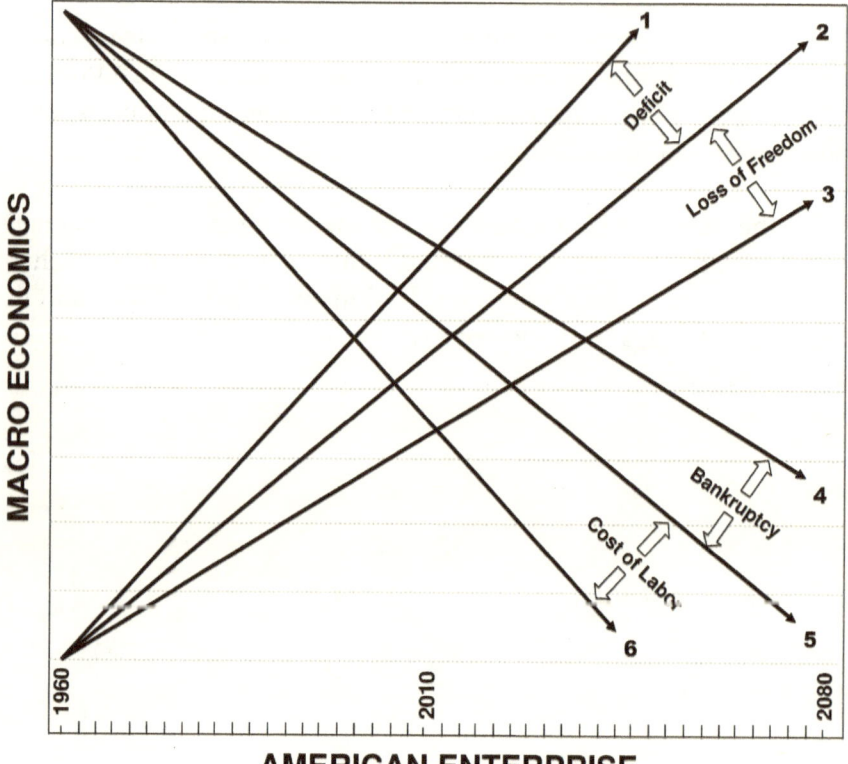

The Monopsony Game:
The economic condition termed Monopsony has a direct impact on enterprise. It drives up the size of government, taxes, and the number of laws passed. At the same rate, it drives down competition and GNP growth rates until they are negative, then destroys employee initiative, work ethic and wage growth. Like a Monopoly, the Monopsony must be broken up or it will break our economy.

LEGEND

1 —— Size of Government
2 —— Taxes
3 —— Laws
4 —— Competition
5 —— GNP Growth
6 —— Work Ethic

ACKNOWLEDGMENTS

The Battelle Institute, for making me aware of the term *monopsony* as applied to health-care economics.

I am indebted to my parents, George and Velma, for giving me the chance to live, love, work, and write. And I am indebted to my wife and her parents, whose lives inspired me to write this book. The untimely and unwarranted deaths of my parents and Shari's mother, Dorotha White, convinced me that there is a better way to live and a better way to die than what they experienced.

I would like to thank my wife, Shari, and our son, Kip, for their support and their belief that we will *remedy eldercide* and *restore elder pride*. Shari is the heart behind this project. Kip is the left brain behind the way we will do it. And I am the right brain, proving it will work. In the process, we are garnering backers, believers, and those that will make it work. So these acknowledgments are only the beginning of the mission that I call the twenty-twenty dream: twenty franchises in twenty major cities, establishing a franchise model of care for the world to follow. The seventy-seven million baby boomers will be the judge, and the health-care profession and health-preservation industry will be the jury. And we hope they will decide that aging is a journey, not a dead end. (Postscript: as a result of the Biggest Bullism in our Washington facility we were forced to sell and put the dream on hold).

I would also like to thank my mentors: Rabbi Hillel Yampol, who taught me persistence in the pursuit of my dreams and let me practice on his playground; Ray Tutwiler, who took a chance on me and then regretted it and then rehired me to help him pursue his dreams; Betty Cornelius of HHS/CMS, who believed in me and promoted my writings and theories in her pursuit of prospective pay for nursing homes; Faye Abdellaha, RN, director of the Division of Long-Term Care and assistant to the Surgeon General of the United States under Richard Nixon, who engaged me to write the white paper for prospective payment for long-term care; Jean Duffy and Elaine Wheaton, chiefs of Medicare claims review at Aetna, who helped me begin the process of developing a deductive library of care-planning models and put me onto Transmittal 262; Keith Hutson, president and CEO of Americana Nursing Centers, who triggered the team concept and quality based on care planning in my brain; Ray Tutwiler, Hillel Yampol, and Terry Penniman, who provided testing grounds for our computerized deductive systems; and over 150 nursing-home facilities that have successfully used a limited version of our deductive case-management systems in their operations.

Duane White, Shari's brother and my brother-in-law, who has been in and out of the business for twenty-six years, always believing in me and my efforts; Kim Lawrence, my daughter, who lent her artistic ability to my marketing materials and seminar offerings; Richard Peck, editor of *Nursing Home Management*, which has published numerous articles that I have written over the years; Ross Reardon, past director of Illinois Health Care Association, who got me into this mess in the first place; Phyllis Vandervelde, Shari's sister, who typed many of the original manuscripts that ended up in the book; Tom Elwood, who was the backbone of the sales force that implements the concepts in the book; Bob Florio and Marty Dickson, my former bankers, and Tom Spread, my current banker, who are believers in elder pride and are helping to fund the future efforts that this book represents; and finally, all the bureaucrats, politicians, consumers, and providers that will make the proposed deductive systems and methods work over the next three decades.

In recognition of the six star staff Shari, Kip and I had at the three All-American Care facilities we salute them as the most caring and dedicated people in health care. We cannot name them all but to Kari Madson and Susie Davis our Director's of Nursing good luck with the new owners . . . we will never forget our love for you, your teams and our patients. We plan to use our experiences to better the plight of long term care.

PART I

AMERICA THE DUTIFUL

(Bound by Rules and Regulations—the Antithesis of Duty Free—"Exempt from the Payment of Certain Local or National duties waived to promote American Enterprise")

DUTY NO. 1—MONOPSONY GAME RULES AND REGS

In 1975, I did a seminar "How to Win the Monopsony Game" for the Illinois Health Care Association on the one-buyer market. Little did I know that we would be losing the monopsony game in 2011 when Obama Care was passed. We now have a government-owned one-buyer market.

The Battelle Institute had offered up this economic phenomena called **monopsony**, a one-buyer market where the buyer (the government) dictates quality and price regardless of profit margins, initially putting small suppliers out of business and encouraging consolidations to capitalize on economies of scale, whereas, in the game of **monopoly**, a single selling force can skew market forces to the point of putting small buyers out of business. Unfortunately, the economies in the service industry are more limited because of the extensive variables and the lack of technology in providing personal-care services.

The marketplace for health care products, since 1966, has slowly become more driven by the availability of the flow of tax revenues than by the natural forces of supply and demand. The reason for this is that the federal government has increasingly become the dominant buyer, which makes the sellers, primarily real estate moguls, more inclined to lobby and less inclined to produce a quality outcome-driven product. In fact, as budgets got higher and margins declined, the suppliers began to rationalize the decline of quality standards unless this dominant buyer was willing to guarantee a profitable price.

The problem generated by this guessing game was that the pricing was based on input units not output units of service as all other businesses are structured. It was focused on income of the providers, not on outcome for the patients. DRGs pay on diagnosis, not on recovery, physicians are paid on RVU's encounters, not wellness;

nursing homes on RUG's assessment of problems, not restorative service resulting in discharges back to the community; OPPS outpatient services based on treatment, not healing; OASIS home care based on visits, not rehabilitation; HOSPICE end of life care based on days of care, not a soft landing.

Unless the buyer collaborates in a consortium with the sellers (not in legal battles but in bipartisan negotiations), an enterprise approach to quality and profits will not be possible. Ultimately, the buyer (that is Obama Care) would have to own the supplier, or there would be no incentive to supply. But if health care were nationalized by the government, as is the VA Health Care system and the postal system, lack of accountability and total ineffectiveness and inefficiencies set in.

The solution, of course, lies in getting the political and the enterprise forces to join together in a privatized collaborative enterprise much like the public utilities. But in this forum, the buyer must deregulate the product so competitive forces can bid for the business based on well-defined products. The inelasticity of this type of market must be dealt with through the influence of quality rather than supply and demand. So the providers of choice would first have to produce products according to set specifications and receive a contracted price, which allows for a margin of profit based on management efficiencies instead of on cost reductions through regulatory enforcement and punitive threats.

In this scenario, productivity and quality become the primary objective. The more efficient providers would then have the best opportunity to establish attractive margins. The buyer must set forth the product specifications and prices in advance. The providers compete against these prices. Cost accounting methodology would be used to determine standards, margins, and prices. The rate setting would create profiles, standard labor inputs, overhead absorption add-ons, and margins for the service component.

The capital component is best based on fair rental values, which convert historical cost to current cost and pay a return based on the standard rental value of the property, plus a working capital investment component. With the investment of capital in the physical plant resolved, the focus must be on the investment in human assets. A commitment needs to be made to develop methods that will measure the production of each individual against a standard of efficiency and pay an incentive when that standard is reached or exceeded.

Organizationally, certain moves must be made if the discipline to exact incentive based productivity is to be implemented. As in the more conventional piecework setting, jobs must be put into set routines. Set tasks must be put in place, time studied and standardized. In health care, this will require an analysis of each product, which converts to specific functions. This specific function becomes a job position, which must be filled. As the position is filled, the task analysis is used to train the worker. Then it will be used to accomplish direct outcomes, for which incentives can be paid.

Health care has not been forced to standardize or functionalize because the major buyer (government) could increase its funding by raising taxes. In 1981, when this leverage switched to budget constraints, product-driven health care entered the market as DRGs (diagnosis-related groups). This was the most significant move in the history of health-care delivery and pricing. Instead of a cost-plus mentality, a fixed price by product was put in place. This impact rippled throughout the health-care marketplace.

Pricing by the buyer based on results in a monopsony is inevitable. The pressures of inadequate funding surfaced in the form of price fixing without regard to the erosive effect on quality. Since the natural force of buyer demand versus supplier desire to profit is missing, the one-buyer market demands more and more for lower and lower marginal prices. The fundamentals of choice are missing. As with embargoes and tariffs, trade will eventually be restrained.

From *The Wealth of Nations* by Adam Smith, the forces of economies are perverted by unnatural restraints. He wrote in 1776:

The exclusive privileges of corporations, statutes of apprenticeship, and all those laws which restrain, in particular employments, the competition to a smaller number than might otherwise go into them, have the same tendency, though in a less degree. They are a sort of enlarged monopolies [monopsonies], and may frequently, for ages together, and in a whole class of employment, keep up [or down] the market price of particular commodities above [or below] the natural price, and maintain [or distain] both the wages of the labor and the profits of the stock employed about them somewhat above [or below] their natural rate. Such enhancements [or erosions] of the market price may last as long as the regulations of police which give occasion to them. The market price of any particular commodity, though it may continue long above, can seldom continue long below its natural price. Whatever part of it was paid below the natural rate, the person whose interest it affected would immediately feel the loss, and would immediately withdraw either so much land, or so much labor, or so much stock from being employed about it, that the quantity brought to market would soon bend more than sufficient to supply the effectual demand. Its market price, therefore, would soon rise to the natural price. This at least would be the case where there was perfect liberty.

(Author to depict the impact of a one-buyer market versus a one-seller market inserts expressions in brackets.)

In our study of health economics in America in the 1990s, we find there is no perfection of liberty. Liberty is dictated by the availability of tax revenues to buy an ever-increasing demand for services. Not only is the liberty distorted, but the perception of product quality is also a major issue because the labor is beginning to be withdrawn if it is not served in its pursuit of economies. Yes, it is a dilemma, but it is also an opportunity to serve a burgeoning market demand with economies of scale, economies of maximum productivity, and economies of responsible cost (input) management in pursuit of profit.

In a monopsony, price follows the productivity levels, not the demand levels. Therefore, productivity measures and cost efficiencies through technology are the only forces left to the supplier in the marketplace, short of legally intimidating and punishing the buyer, which further erodes margins.

Cost accounting in health care, until the advent of product definition (DRGs), was so rudimentary that it functioned strictly on averages. The concept of pricing and cost accounting using the patient day as the unit of production proved that averages are for average results. The following is an illustration of the impact of being average: the guy has a bare foot in the bucket of ice-cold water and the other in a bucket of boiling hot water, and on average, he should feel great. But in reality, relegating everything to average is wasting away valuable resources on average to below-average work ethic and acceptable low quality.

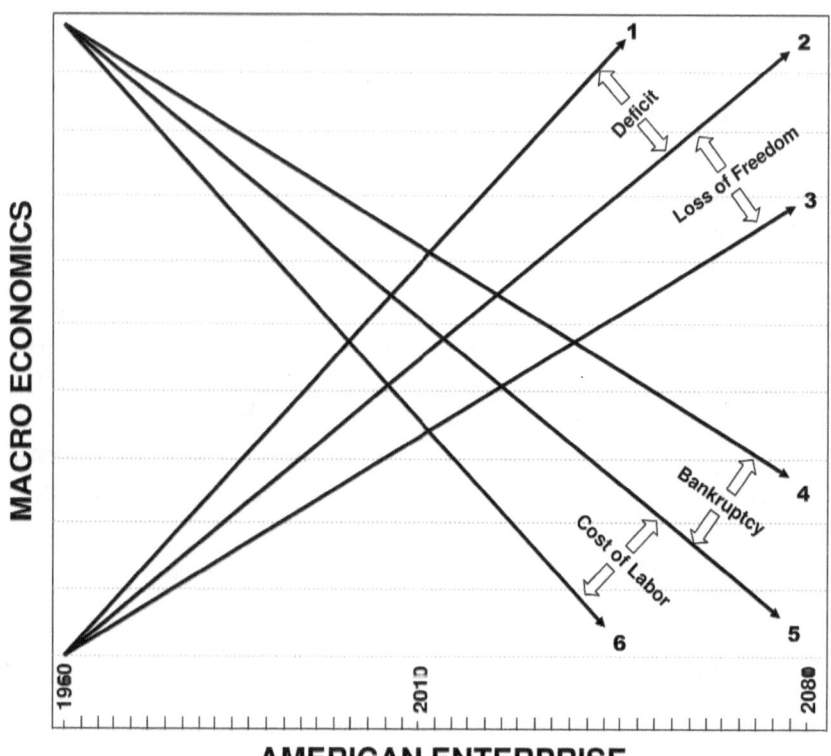

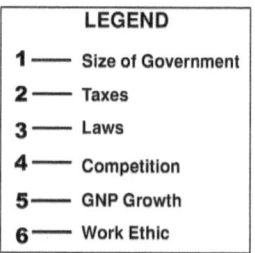

The Monopsony Game:
The economic condition termed Monopsony has a direct impact on enterprise. It drives up the size of government, taxes, and the number of laws passed. At the same rate, it drives down competition and GNP growth rates until they are negative, then destroys employee initiative, work ethic and wage growth. Like a Monopoly, the Monopsony must be broken up or it will break our economy.

Cost accounting for specific products focuses on specifics, not averages. The only way to deal with increasing labor costs per unit of production is to isolate, define, and arrive at standards for efficiency and productivity and set incentives for the same. Again, we must understand the wealth of our nation so we can understand and capitalize on the wealth of individuals. Again, Adam Smith's intellect states:

> The demand for those who live by wages, therefore, necessarily increases with the increase of revenue and stock of every country, and cannot possibly increase without it. The increase of revenue and stock is the increase in natural wealth [health]. The demand for those who live by wages, therefore, naturally increases with the increase of national wealth [health], and cannot possibly increase without it. (Brackets are again inserted by author to connect wealth and health.)

In other words, the relationship of individual wealth and national wealth are the roots of a high standard of living but by the natural process where the wealth of the individual converts to products that create the wealth (health) of America. In this sense (cents), the labor component of the health of our nation creates the key to success in quantities as well as qualities.

But this line of thought gets us back to a detailed definition of products in terms of the labor component, first and foremost, which carries with it the flow of other resources (food, supplies, overhead factors for space, equipment, taxes, etc.). These are the elements of cost accounting. All, and I repeat, all successful businesses that survive the test of time and its natural swings have a well-defined profile of its products and what they cost, down to the finest detail, compared to what they should cost, in an efficient setting, to be produced in the form that meets the acceptable standards of quality. If this definition does not exist, management is not managing the business. Instead, the outside forces of health economics (surveyors, legal action labor unions, bankruptcy court, and receivership) are managing the business.

This penny-wise, pound-foolish phenomenon has been attributed to mom-and-pop business methods. If the shoe fits, you must wear it until you change it or wear it out. My suggestion is to implement cost-accounting procedures before someone else owns your shoe. Again, Adam Smith's insight gives us clarity:

> We are more industrious than our forefathers; because in the present times the funds destined for the maintenance of industry, are much greater in proportion to those which are likely to be employed in the maintenance of idleness. Our ancestors were idle for want of sufficient encouragement to industry. It is better, says the proverb, to play for nothing than work for nothing. In mercantile and manufacturing towns where the inferior ranks of people are chiefly maintained by the employment of capital, they are in general industrious, sober and thriving.

In the health-care economy, the labor component (clearly 75 percent of the cost to produce) must be efficiently employed if the individual is to accumulate wealth (profit) and the nation is to profit. Cost accounting clearly puts this in perspective because it clearly defines standards of production, which becomes the definition of efficiency. Then it must measure actual results against the standards and pay compensation based on the attainment of the efficiency standards.

In more definitive products, the engineered drawing of the product is the starting point for the cost accountant to lay out standards for the following components:

- Labor
- Material usage
- Overhead absorption
- Setting of margins based on market factors
- Profit forecasts utilizing sales forecasts and budgets

In health care, the products defied definition until the federal government decided it would buy products instead of esoteric services. The definition became the disease group being treated. The diagnosis determined the treatment regimens and the utilization of cost resources, so why shouldn't it constitute the product cost profile and pricing mechanism? Since health care was operating in a monopsonistic market, the buyer set the process in motion by dictating what it would buy according to a diagnostic group and not according to per diems (which are daily averages at best). This shortcut averaging process did not put health care in the competitive, cost-conscious, mercantile business. It allowed health care to continue to hide from cost-management responsibilities. It further institutionalized all processes and allowed regulators and bureaucrats to dictate the reimbursement levels. It did not responsibly deal with product definition, labor standards, efficiency measurements, productivity levels, and ultimately, incentive salary methods.

Congress and its ineffective committee, subcommittee institutional structure, allow the conglomerates to gobble up the providers pursuing profits based on illness rather than incentives for pursuing wellness. The Department of Health and Human Services and its gestapo agency, CMS, ignore the economies of enterprise for sake of control for budgetary purposes. What is the solution? Privatization of health care based on outcome to create income and quality of health-care priorities that are prevention and preservation of the human genome.

Since the salary costs at best are only 20 percent variable in the health care business, productivity and cost-management methods must be mandated for change from a monopsony to an enterprise model. As such systems are implemented, a certain portion of salary costs will become directly variable, with increases in efficiency and productivity. These costs that have been semivariable or fixed, because it takes a certain base staff to cover the operation regardless of patient acuities, can now be related to production and outcome management. In this manner, patient acuities can be defined in cost terms, because they are now related to the restorative regimens and standard therapeutic approaches.

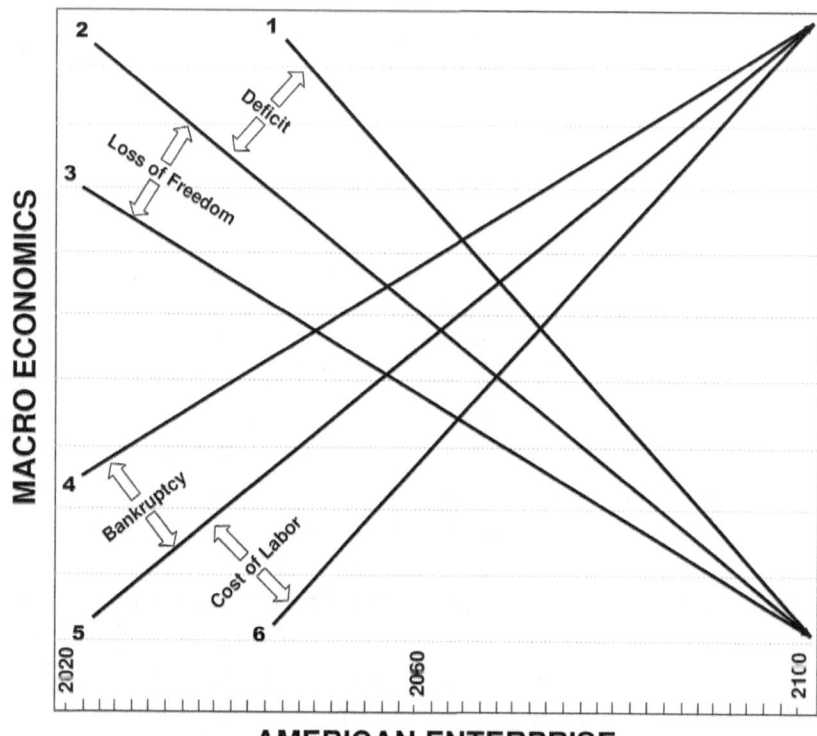

Using the productivity measures and the incentive methods factored into the standard product models, the above natural economies can be attained. Efficiency improvements will impact margins and price. A privatized marketplace needs to be dictating price so most of the improvements will result, in the short run, in better margins (higher profits or lower losses). In this arena, the need to use negative legal pressures to force the price up is supplanted by positive management techniques. Ultimately, this is the only realistic way the sellers can negotiate better prices with the dominant single (mono) buyer. That buyer also has unlimited legal manpower and an enforcement posse (OIG and IRS) to use as the ultimate seek-and-destroy tactic.

At the same time, management must look to the smaller market segments for margins. But with a more cost-effective delivery system in place, the pricing of other markets can be more competitive. Self-pay (private) is everyone's pursuit and no one's captive, and amazingly, it is not the most profitable approach. Because of the lack of sophistication in the methods of costing products, it is assumed that private-pay pricing subsidizes government buyers. In reality, the profit margin, which contributes the most to the operation, is the quality of the product and not the payer contribution to that margin. Until the products are defined and segmented for cost accounting, it is not possible to analyze profitability, its impact on pricing, and the elasticity to the buyer. The add-ons, the options, the accessories, the specialized services, and the ancillaries all contribute a substantial "piece of the action!"

The utility of the product then enters the formula. What carries more utility to the buyer: the accommodation (room and board), the treatment, or the outcome?

Of course, it is the therapy treatment that produces an improvement in functioning that also carries the leverage for margin, but it is the psycho/social and spiritual restorative services that enable discharge to the community. It contributes more to the value of the patient's care than the room/board and treatment for the sake of treatment. The real business is the restorative care product, not the hotel-type service. The hotel component is the bait, the loss leader.

Utility of the product, in every business, carries the value, and value carries the supply and price. The price carries cost and margin. It is then up to management to balance productivity with demand and cost with price, so the margin is maximized. Management must also decide whether to use loss leaders (low-margin products) to attract higher margin options and if it will make its acceptable returns on investment from quantitative methods, qualitative standards, or a combination of both.

But no matter how you stratify the market, value carries the widest margin, as utility is the quality of the product merchandised at the most competitive price. In this way, the well-managed business is successful at costing its product, pricing for margins based on utility, and managing productivity. These basic economic theories are relentless in a one-buyer market because the mono buyer sets the price of 75 percent of the market. So the successful healthcare provider is one that accomplishes efficiency in delivering its government-purchased products and uses those margins to streamline and manage its smaller market segments. In this arena, if a provider is well managed, it has the competitive edge in the remaining 25 percent of its market.

Americana Nursing Homes, under Keith Hutson's tutelage, used this pricing strategy in the 1970s to capture private market share by offering maximum utility (therapy) that could be paid for by Medicare (utility and pricing strategy). This approach saved private resources for better accommodations with the luxuries of the home environment. Today the smart operators of nursing homes must still use these strategies if they expect to capture a lasting share of the smaller market segments (HMOs, insurance contracts, Veterans Administration).

The strategy of "we are only going to admit private pay" will achieve limited success as labor costs continue to rise and naturally drive up prices to private pay. That segment is now basically limited to the affluent, who are in a minority in our society. As in hospitals, costs will rise to the point where mass funding must be used by the affluent, or they basically waste their savings on low-utility products. Insurance funding became a necessity in order for hospitals to provide a quality product. (Individual resources shrink in the purge of high-cost labor and with low-performance technologies.)

It is a distinct likelihood that private-pay funding for nursing home care will disappear, as it did in the hospital business. In anticipation of this trend, the intelligent health-care provider will focus its marketing on saving the private dollar, by billing someone else, before they waste the private dollar. It is this mentality that requires a product approach be developed with quality replacing source of payment as the main objective.

Given that higher utility can be purchased from a cost-efficient provider, pricing strategies can be used to attract managed care resources through "more for the money" offerings. Over a period or time, this "attrition" strategy can reduce the provider's dependence on cost-based government-funded programs by shifting the control to mutually owned private health-insurance entities that are owned by their members. Then reimbursement can be from individual self-health insurance funding trusts. *Shift* of the paradigm to withholding from each employee's paycheck for their use in managing their own health-care needs and prevention and preservation of their most valuable asset, their minds and bodies. Shift also assigns the responsibility for health care to each individual, not just to the healthy paying for the bad habits of the unhealthy.

Health economics has quality as its bottom line. A manager (with a heart) in this business is compelled to be sensitive to business as well as compassionate to the patient's need to "manage with head and heart." The pinch comes as labor costs and then competition bite away at the profit. Then management is the margin. What would you, as a manager of a present-day health facility, do if profit were disappearing? Here are your options:

1. Cut costs (most elementary)
2. Raise prices
3. Raise volume of ancillaries
4. Raise productivity
5. Cut semi-variable cost
6. Charge for more specific services
7. Increase markets
8. Improve quality
9. Increase advertising
10. Remove credit restrictions

11. Give discounts
12. Cut quality
13. Cut fixed costs, relocate, or cut and run
14. Change product lines
15. Diversify
16. Merge/consolidate with another facility (horizontal integration)
17. Merge with a supplier or hospitals (vertical integration)
18. Fill beds

In the past, the mom-and-pop approach would have been to strictly fill beds with private-pay patients and keep costs down. The owner's mentality (particularly if they were absentee owners) was to make money first and worry about social responsibilities if they could afford it. The chain operations merely pyramided this erosive philosophy. Even many of the nonprofit operations succumbed to this warehouse approach. The state of affairs now has necessitated the mono buyer to intimidate the seller into providing quality regardless of cost. More and more regulations abound.

Of course, the solution is in the management of revenue (production and pricing) and labor while eliminating waste and theft of supplies. Consolidation of resources by chain operations merely adds overhead unless a decentralized, franchised approach is followed. Therefore, the well-managed business would select from above the following alternatives:

No. 3. *Raise volume of ancillary restorative services.* Restorative ancillaries represent options that carry utilitarian value and higher margins.

No. 4. *Raise productivity.* Efficiency of labor and elimination of excess capacity are the major contributors to margins in a monopsony.

No. 6. *Charge for more specific services.* Specific and well-defined products provide higher opportunities for marginal profits.

No. 8. *Improve quality.* Markets demanding more quality will skew to a product commitment.

No. 11. *Give discounts.* Government buyers should get volume discounts because they dictate the prices they pay. They should also get discounts on the pricing of ancillaries for improving the health of the covered lives.

The remainder of the options should be studied, but only to understand why they will not work in the current monopsony health-care market.

No. 1. *Cut variable costs in health care.* The blind obsession of cutting variable cost to the breakeven point turns even the best facility into a ghetto. The need for labor and adequate supplies almost puts fixed costs at 90 percent of total. This leaves little margin or categorical cost cutting, except labor efficiency and productivity.

No. 2. *Raise prices to private pay.* The pass-through of 100 percent of the labor cost increases to 40 percent of the caseload merely drives more of the census toward financial indecency. (They run out of money and go on the Medicaid welfare / low-margin rolls.)

No. 5. *Cut semi-variable costs for fringe benefits, building maintenance, volume purchasing, and management personnel.* Again, it is shortsighted to just cut costs to gain financial stability. In health care, there are few, if any, semi-variable costs because of the regulated influences, which dictate cost patterns.

No. 7. *Increase markets.* The fact that health care is primarily a one-buyer market doesn't lend itself to fancy market segmentation and marketing. Austerity is the negative incentive.

No. 9. *Increase advertising.* It's a waste of valuable resources to compete for dwindling private markets that respond to a quality product more than they respond to hype.

No. 10. *Remove credit restrictions.* If the buyer was being frightened away because of inhibiting credit restrictions, this move might work. But in health care, credit is only a factor with private pay. And since they are expected to pay in advance and generally do, this credit-relief tactic won't do any good. The challenge is to qualify more and more of the market for disability and Medicaid coverage after the Medicare money runs out.

No. 12 *Cut quality.* The typical "people warehouser" facility will cut quality as they cut staffing levels in an attempt to maintain margins, in spite of escalating labor costs.

No. 13. *Cut fixed costs, relocate, or cut and run.* Many inefficient, poorly managed facilities will sell out to pyramiders or franchisers of management systems. The days of mom-and-pop management, even in chain operations, has been gone since the consolidation sprees in the 1990s (as it was in hospitals in the 1980s). Economies of scale are still touted in the twenty-first century with poor quality and shallow promises of quality and outcome management.

No. 14. *Change product.* Some providers will strive to avoid heavy-care patients and will succumb to low-census levels. The next generation of ownership will be able to acquire such facilities for residential housing or step down from subacute care units. The smaller size will put most existing facilities out of the health-care business. Their future may lie in day care, respite care, assisted living (boarding care), and short-term crisis care.

No. 15. *Diversify or die.* This is happening to hospitals, but they have capital. Your typical nursing home has not accumulated enough capital to buy the time to diversify. So they will die, as did small banks, hospitals, and savings and loans. Quality will die along with mom-and-pop owners.

No. 16. *Merge/consolidate with another facility (horizontal integration).* Horizontal integration in the 1970s and 1980s had been a diabolical disaster. The chains offered economies of scale, economies of expertise, and economies of management—none of which materialized. They merely centralized poor management methods that made performance worse instead of better. Any move to consolidate, if it does not recognize that wisdom must lie in the authority of the line worker, eventually destroys effectiveness. The chains need to franchise proven management methods and systems and give guidance in implementing proven methods. But they have, instead, centralized authoritarian, ivory-tower approaches to a personal-service business, which, by its very nature, requires decentralized authority and incentives to go with the extreme amount of responsibility. (Life and death rest in the daily regimen of the nursing-home worker, and some try to delegate such responsibility to low-paid workers who get directives from absent/inept order givers.)

No. 17. *Merge with a supplier or hospitals (vertical integration).* This has also been ineffective because it compounds inefficiency even though it should smooth the flow of patients through the continuum of care. The other units in the continuum at this time in history are also only marginally successful. They also have to improve their management methods.

No. 18. *Fill beds.* Hospitals deduced in the 1970s and 1980s that they could survive if they filled empty med surgical beds with longer-term care patients. Nursing homes deduced they could thrive by displacing beds occupied by welfare recipients with the "well walking wealthy." What a shortsighted group of mismanagers! These dreams of winning the health-care monopsony game should not give the smart businessperson quite an opportunity. But which approach do you choose?

- ➢ Profit or quality product?
- ➢ Quality product or profit?
- ➢ Which comes first?
- ➢ Can we have both?

My position is that we must have both. Society, our primary and only buyer, won't stand for less. There lies the opportunity for a franchise. We can conquer the influences of a one-buyer market with the following:

- A franchise model of innovative service products.
- Use cost-accounting methodology to maximize efficiency and effectiveness:
  o The outcome pricing approach.

- o The restorative marketing technique.
- o The quality-based production schedules, including productivity measures and incentives.
- All of the above supported by policies, protocols, and procedures by which the resources are managed pursuing outcomes rather than treatment.
- A computer system that monitors results and documents performance by patient and episode.

Doing so, we will have managed productivity in delivering a quality product and produce acceptable margins for reinvestment and replenishing of capital assets through economizing on quality and volume, not through monopsonized margins. The systematic franchise of health care will best serve the privatized monopsony.

The for-profit franchise of health care will become a bigger factor because it allows the employee to share in the profits (through incentives), which can build momentum in offering further quality programs for maximized revenues and maximized profit. This is an investment in the most valuable asset in health care: human value!

Winning the monopsony game will require that our government relinquish control of the natural forces of enterprise and stop the bully pulpit that now exists with Congress and bureaucrats dictating academic solutions that cannot be implemented efficiently and effectively so our health-care policies and procedures can breathe life into the unhealthy and unfundable lifestyles and *bad* habits of Americans. Privatize, economize, systemize the processes, and get enforcement out of the way. The biggest bully does inhibit our use of China's funding of our debt-driven health-care economy.

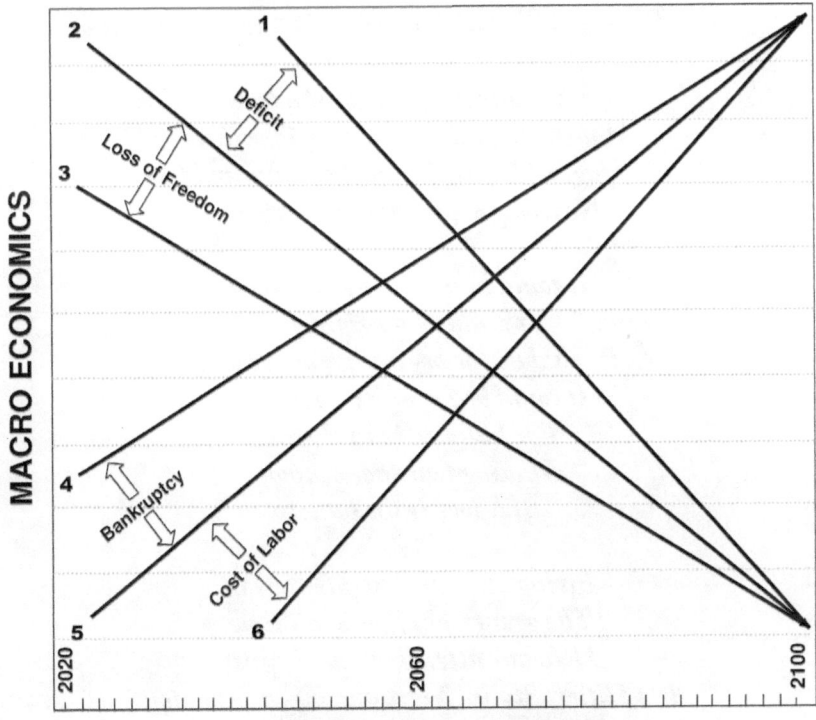

Winning The Monopsony Game:
This Monopsony Game can be won, if and when the voters decide to slow the growth of government; control taxation; remove unneeded laws that produce more resources for wage growth for the working Americans; improve small business employee's morale; and allow for the benefits of competition, such as creativity, technology and profitability. Thereby reducing the deficits and labor costs, while getting rid of laws that inhibit small business and GNP growth and solidifying America's position of economic leadership in the world, would create a "Win-Win" for everyone.

LEGEND
1 —— Size of Government
2 —— Taxes
3 —— Laws
4 —— Competition
5 —— GNP Growth
6 —— Work Ethic

DUTY NO. 2—WHO IS THE BIGGEST BULLY (in China's Shop)?

THE BIGGEST BULLY (We All Are the Victims)

The bully hides in the shadows
Making the mission misery for others
Lurking in the memories of tyrants and foes
No thought of sisters or brothers

It could be an enemy or friend
It could be a neighbor
It could be the beginning or the end
It could be far off or next door
The bully talks in threats
Making fear the weapon
And words the bullets

Firing on your daughter or son
The greatest bullies of all time
Hold our attention and disgust
As a Hitler, Stalin, Mao, and big government
Forgetting in God we trust
By using technology against us

When you hear the story
Of another event gone wrong
Remember that old glory
Expects us bullied to be strong
By taking on the shadow in disguise
Exposing their intent
By challenging their lies
With proof and descent

Failing Government Taketh Away

No bully has the right
To take away the freedom
Of thought, effort, and insight
Making us all deaf and dumb
The biggest bully of them all
Is the government that controls
Our thoughts, efforts, and right to fail
Degrading our hearts and souls

So stand up for your rights
Or you will fall for anything
For freedom only comes from fights
Against bullies that hold us by our wings
Because they are in the bully pulpit
That allows them to fabricate
Distort and assert allegations that commit
A disregard for due process, as in Jersey Bridgegate

Wake up America, for as reason sleeps
Big Brother Congress wins with fear they reap
Better yet, while the President creeps
Our hopes and fears won't keep

The biggest bully from trampling China
Russia, India, and Japan
In this arrogant world of America
Because they can

—Jerry Rhoads, victim and author

This book is written to highlight the battle we wage with ourselves. Pogo says, "We searched for the enemy, and it is us." America is in the hands of a few waging a war of money with the freedoms of the American enterprising worker and the aging baby boomers demanding their rights to Medicare. My feeling is that big government eventually turns us all into liars and cheats because survival becomes the instinct, not peace or love or patriotism. We are lost to the fear of reprisal, fear of losing our job, fear of being on the street, fear of dying poor, fear of having someone else make our decisions, when the only thing we should fear is fear itself. We have lawmakers working hard to bury our freedom to participate in the American dream with more and more laws.

In the following pages, I am compelled by experience to educate the enterprising public of the tactics being used to thwart change and deprive the private sector of their rights to fail and protect themselves. Do you have to be an attorney to understand that government is more than laws and regulations? If you do, then we are all destined to be dumbed down to a level of being the victim being protected from ourselves.

Politicians and political pundits—who intellectually spout theory as facts and facts as the domain of the Congress, the elite, the media, and never putting forth the voice of the silent majority—are using fear to dumb down enterprising Americans. CNN, Fox News, MSNBC, conservative radio, liberal leanings of the celebrities are not reporting the depth or breadth of America's decline. They are, in fact, the beneficiary of the hardworking, enterprising majority who do not have a voice. I, as an unknown nonintellectual, will be accused of being unqualified politically, negative on America and idealistic on foreign affairs. Right up front, I want to state that America, in my view, is the greatest example of capital-driven enterprise ever known to man and woman, including the British Empire, the past German and current Chinese versions. However, all good things come to an end unless there is revitalization of the principles that got us here.

So much of this book is based on factual data and statistics gleaned over a number of years as I wrote manuscripts regarding the need for political and government reform to ensure we worship enterprise rather than institutionalized money. In my research, I found that certain individuals have contributed to contrasting opinions that became movements and did solve social and economic problems. Why because they were, first of all, superior leaders and, second, dedicated to preserving the past and conserving the future. Margaret Thatcher and Ronald Reagan were two such leaders of conservatism that inspired me to write this book. Because it proposes that we restore old American-style enterprise that evolved out of the slave-supported plantations and Aquarian-farm communities, into the cities of industrial blue-collar workers and profit-seeking white-collar business owners, serving our academic universities and institutions. But now, such academic laws and PhD regulators are stifling our effectiveness to utilize what we learn from the universities and colleges without allowing the private sector to manage the implementation. Because of this infringement of big institutional government on individual creativity and freedom, for the sake of control by the bigger and bigger universities and institutions, we are hampered by our own incompetence. To alter this "Rome is burning" mentality, we have to have a balance of the private sector and public institutions, or we will evolve into a world of continued declining initiative and more divorces of thought and families. We need to realize that reality does not create us—we create reality with common-sense solutions to problems, not just debating political issues. We can learn much from Margaret Thatcher and Ronald Reagan in their campaign to have "government protect us, not run our lives," as opposed to what Karl Marx stood for in his *Communist Manifesto*.

Margaret Thatcher (1925–2013), Prime Minister of England (1979–1990)

- "There is no such thing as society: there are individual men and women, and there are families".
- "If you just set out to be liked, you would be prepared to compromise on anything at any time, and you would achieve nothing".
- "It is not the creation of wealth that is wrong, but the love of money for its own sake".

Margaret Thatcher dealt with similar economic problems in England that America now has, *as leader of the Conservative Party from 1975 to 1990 and prime minister from 1979 to 1990.* She was an advocate of privatizing State-owned industries and utilities, reforming trade unions, lowering taxes, and reducing social expenditure across the board. Thatcher's policies succeeded in reducing inflation, but unemployment dramatically increased during her years in power. However, it was her leadership that directed the British away from socialism back to capitalizing on enterprising workers for the sake of the country's future. The movie the *Iron Lady* did not give justice to Margaret's influence in making one of the most significant socioeconomic changes of all time. Since she died in April 2013, we are not going to have her counsel or involvement in world economics or enterprise, so in America, in her memory, we must challenge big government and the socialist form of democracy at all times. She and Ronald Reagan had a bond based on America's philosophy that the individual makes the country and that the country does not make the individual. It is such leaders we have to revere, and we should not be deterred by spin doctors and lobbyists.

Ronald Reagan (1911–2004), President of the United States (1981–1989)

- "Entrepreneurs and their small enterprises are responsible for almost all the economic growth in the United States."
- "Government exists to protect us from each other. Where government has gone beyond its limits is in deciding to protect us from ourselves".
- "Government does not solve problems; it subsidizes them".
- "Government's first duty is to protect the people, not run their lives".

Ronald Reagan, on his eight-year watch, was following a one-term Democratic president in Jimmie Carter, who pushed American businesses to the brink with his 23 percent Keynesian prime rate of interest to quell record inflation and destroyed the savings and loan business forever. President Reagan was lucky to inherit Alan Greenspan as the chairman of the Federal Reserve Bank, who, by chance, had ultraconservative libertarian leanings. President Reagan also engaged Fr. Arthur Laffer, who became the father of supply-side economics, as his chief advisor on taxation, who then, with a Republican House, put trickledown economics into action. With the interest rates and monetary system in check and taxes being cut, small businesses were relieved of debt and created products and profits at a record pace. Unemployment declined, but still the deficits rose. Unfortunately, Bush, Sr. following Reagan, who was a civil servant, not entrepreneurial, who famously said "Read my lips: no tax increases" then proceeded to increase taxes to his demise.

Then Bill Clinton, the smooth-talking salesman, had the country in developmental mode until the high-tech bubble burst. All the while, conservatives on the Republican side acquiesced to a staggering war budget and a fiscal depression under Bush Jr. selling out to a protectionist government pursuing a one-world version of liberty. Then Obama, a liberal constitutional professor and street attorney, rides in on his oratory ability, right in the middle of a depression, and worsens it with a misguided $700 billion stimulus package for the bailout of large banks and big business, financed by China, and imposes the biggest entitlement of all time: Obama Care, which may well be the demise of the great American enterprise and its 77 million retiring, unhealthy baby boomers.

To quote Ronald Reagan again, "Above all, we must realize that no arsenal, or arsenals of the world, is so formidable as the will and moral courage of free men and women. It is a weapon our adversaries in today's world do not have."

Karl Marx (1818–1883), the author who wrote the *Communist Manifesto* in 1848, put forth his ten steps necessary to destroy capitalism in a free-enterprise system and replace it with a system of omnipotent government power, so as to affect a communist socialist state. Unfortunately, many Americans are being transformed into a communist state of mind, by myths, fraud, and deception under the color of law by their own politicians, Republican and Democratic Parties alike. Karl Marx, in creating the Communist Manifesto, designed the ten planks ***as a test*** to determine whether a society is becoming communist or not. The ten *planks* stated in the Communist Manifesto (and some of their American counterparts [in parentheses]) are the following:

1. Abolition of private property and the application of all rents of land to public purposes (imminent domain lost to federalism of property)
2. A heavy progressive or graduated income tax (graduated taxation on adjusted gross income)
3. Abolition of all rights of inheritance (inheritance or death tax)
4. Confiscation of the property of all emigrants and rebels (laws preventing aliens from owning property)
5. Centralization of credit in the hands of the State, by means of a national bank with State capital and an exclusive monopoly (the Federal Reserve Bank)
6. Centralization of the means of communications and transportation in the hands of the State (FCC)
7. Extension of factories and instruments of production owned by the State, the bringing into cultivation of waste lands, and the improvement of the soil generally in accordance with a common plan (EPA, EEOC)
8. Equal liability of all to labor; establishment of industrial armies, especially for agriculture (NLRB and unionization of labor)
9. Combination of agriculture with manufacturing industries, gradual abolition of the distinction between town and country, by a more equitable distribution of population over the country (corporate conglomerates with farm quotas and subsidies)
10. Free education for all children in public schools; abolition of children's factory labor in its present form; combination of education with industrial production (public education funded by property taxes, gambling taxes, Powerball, and lotto)

The **progressives (politicians)** of the twenty-first century who seem to believe in the *socialistic* and *neocommunist* concepts, especially those who pass more and more laws implementing those ideas, are contradicting their oath of office and to the Constitution of the United States of America. None are more hopelessly enslaved as those who falsely believe they are free.

THEY ARE COLONIZED AND LIONIZED BULLIES.

What does this do for our relationships around the world:

- o   The China Shop … with a market share of 19% Population 1.351 billion (2012)

- The USA Shop … with a market share of 25% with only 4% of the World Population of 319 million (2014)
  - o   The Indian Shop … 1.2 billion 17%
  - o   The Russian Shop 143 million … 2%
  - o   The Japan Shop 126.6 million … 1.7%
  - o   The Mexico Shop 117.4 million … 1.5%
  - o   The Canadian Shop 35.2 million … .5%
  - o   The South American Shop 399.2 million … 5.5%
  - o   The Great Britain Shop … 63.7 million … .9%
  - o   The French Shop … 64.3 million … .9%
  - o   The Rest of the World Shop … 3.500 billion 50%
  - o   The total population = 7.1 billion

What is the catch to the monopsony game rules?

Catch 23 is the exhausting of administrative remedies that are required before you can plead your case in court. It eliminates government accountability with no due process of law due to indemnification and no appeal rights. If you remember catch 22 (the Joseph Heller novel looks into the experiences of Yossarian and the other airmen in the camp and their attempts to keep their sanity in order to fulfill their service requirements so that they can return home; the phrase "catch 22" is a problematic situation for which the only solution is denied by a circumstance inherent in the problem or by a rule), it has become a symbolic word in the English language signifying being in an endless bureaucratic maze going nowhere fast.

"You mean there's a catch?"

"Sure there's a catch", Doc Daneeka replied. "Catch-22. Anyone who wants to get out of combat duty isn't really crazy and if they are not crazy then they can handle combat."

There was only one catch and that was Catch-22, which specified that a concern for one's own safety in the face of dangers that were real and immediate was the process of a rational mind. Or was crazy and could be grounded. All he had to do was ask; and as soon as he did, he would no longer be crazy and would have to fly more missions. Or would be crazy to fly more missions and sane if he didn't, but if he was sane, he had to fly them. If he flew them, he was crazy and didn't have to; but if he didn't want to, he was sane and had to. Yossarian was moved very deeply by the absolute simplicity of this clause of Catch-22 and let out a respectful whistle.

Our situation in the nursing-home business is a catch 23 since it is not only impossible to get justice because you must exhaust your administrative remedies, but it is impossible to satisfy the requirements that enable the defendant to get due process. It has to be handled by an attorney licensed in that state, because an individual cannot represent a company in hearings and court unless they are a licensed attorney, and licensed attorneys charge $250 to $1,000 per hour, making it prohibitive to even attempt what is called due process of law. Even when the agency violates the Administrative Procedure Act by being arbitrary and capricious with their actions, you cannot challenge their allegations unless you have deep pockets, and then the process drags out for years before you can get to a court of law. In between, you have departmental appeals and an administrative law judge who works for the government to stall and disregard the need for due process to hold the agency accountable.

For example, say there is a rule that a health-care provider perform CPR (cardiopulmonary resuscitation) on anyone that does not have a written form stating they don't want to be resuscitated. If they do not perform CPR, it is a violation chargeable as patient abuse and penalized at the rate of $6,000 per day until they decide you now can comply with this interpretive guideline.

Another example is using security videos against the provider as an entrapment of situations that are related to defending the provider rather than penalizing them or requiring that the provider self-report incidences that incriminate them and result in punitive fines, holds on new admissions, holds on Medicare and Medicaid funding and criminal allegations.

Throughout *The Biggest Bully*, we will establish how unfettered this process is and how the ripple affect not only hurts due process it hurts the patient care because of the loss of funds, it hurts the staff because of damaged morale, it hurts communities because of the loss of business, it hurts owners who have risked their money in good faith, and it hurts the country because enterprise cannot function when the risks outweigh the rewards.

For the first time in my life, I truly wanted to have a law degree so I could establish that the biggest bully lawmakers are getting me and I have no way to hold them accountable or pay my fee. My fee is to make a profit, pay taxes to pay the judges and attorneys that are in charge so they will free me to be enterprising and profitable in spite of the lawmakers. But the attorney's fees are so expensive I cannot afford to appeal.

Who would want to independently own a business that assigns all responsibility, reasonable or not, to the owner and all authority unreasonable or not, to the buyer? ... the classic definition of Monopsony:

For example: the Federal and State regulators have full access to any and all records of the targeted nursing home without warrants, due process or even proving they are not themselves sex offenders ... all the while requiring that we check all who cross the threshold to be back round checked, strip searched and interrogated.

For example: anyone can call the 800 number of the Department of Inspections and Appeals and make any and all allegations about the care, the owners, the work conditions, the handling of patient accidents and incidences, the environment, the employee conditions, the physical plant, the exterior, the driveway, unfair practices, falls, injuries, etc. Most times the complaints are from former employees terminated for good reason. Some are from families or patients who did not approach management but just pick up the phone and incriminate because of course nursing homes are "guilty until proven innocent" regardless of severity, truth, consequences, or reputation. It is open season for the "gotcha" system that has been in place for 30+ years and has made the conditions worse not better.

For example: the owner cannot run the business unless they have a bachelor's degree regardless of proven ability and investment. The owner has to be a licensed Administrator to run their own business. Then hire someone less competent to be the boss while the owner still has all the risk.

For example: the surveyor can come on site without announcing why they are there, treat the staff like criminals and start demanding any and all records, interview anyone they choose to intimidate digging as much dirt as possible to justify fines and putative actions.

For example: recently one of our facilities had a noncompliant patient loan a nurse aide $5.00 for gas. The staff person was terminated and had not repaid the loan. The Activity Director replaced the $5.00 but the incident was considered patient abuse by a team leader who turned it in as "reportable". The terminated employee was brought back and repaid the $5.00. This resulted in a full scale assault on the staff, the owner and the patient involved treating it as a major offense.

For example: this same noncompliant patient was involved in numerous violent incidences but was given more credibility in interviews than the staff, the owner and the other witnesses. He had been the source of three of the four complaints being investigated over a two week period. He accused the owner of swearing at him and accusing him of losing his temper when in fact the owner called the police because of the vulgarity and violent behavior. Of course the interrogation was of the owner not the perpetrator.

For example: annual surveys are the bane of any nursing home because you are held hostage for two weeks and never know how you are doing or what they are conjuring up for your 2567 F-tags that usually result in putative action and fines. Fear runs nursing homes not the owners or managers. It has for 35 years making the circumstances worse because it has forced the small independent owners out of the business. How can negative enforcement get positive creative results ... it never has and never will.

So why would any self-respecting business person want to be --

1. Criticized with no due process for defending themselves
2. Vandalized for petty mistakes
3. Terrorized for ineffective rules
4. Scrutinized and second guessed on every incident
5. Chastised for thinking differently
6. Penalized because the regulators have the authority to convict without due process

The solutions proposed in this book are for collaboration not more intimidation. For cooperation with the private sector not more academic rules and standards. For individualized payment for results not average payment for wasted resources.

Count successes not mistakes. How many patients are restored and discharged back to the community, instead of perfect diaper changing and pill passing on time. How many patients are out of wheelchairs, instead of alarms on wheel chairs to trigger falls not prevent them. How many patients participate in small group classes and clubs, instead of large group bingo games and boring entertainment. How many staff are getting help on improving their skills, instead of rehiring continually for replacements. How many patients are prevented from being re-hospitalized and/or sent to the ER inappropriately, instead of using observation days to prevent the patients from getting their Medicare benefits. How many family members are involved in the care planning and discharge planning, instead of uninvolved families and money grubbing as the family power of attorney representative to keep the social security and disability check.

The change in payment must relate to add services and a quality incentive payment such as Illinois had in the 1980s:

SIX STARS TO PROVEN QUALITY

The only system that has been developed that works is the Illinois six star system for skilled nursing facilities (after having had a point system for twenty years) (I refer to this in my books). It was implemented with my help in the 1980's by the Department of Public Health and was called QUIP (quality incentive program). It measures outcome results not input units of mistakes and inaccurate metrics for quality of care and life. The six stars was an annual re-enforcement survey in six areas of outcome where the surveyors measured performance on those criteria that could be defined as contributing to the patients' welfare and functionality. It was collaborative and far exceeded the success of our current enforcement mentality.

- First star = care planning and staff effectiveness
- Second star = documentation of attaining goals for problems
- Third star = family involvement and satisfaction
- Fourth star = Community and volunteer involvement
- Fifth star = productive activities and psycho/social programming
- Sixth star = discharge planning

The corresponding reimbursement system then paid for the add-on programs of restorative care that generated the six star results. It then paid an economic incentive for each star earned and paid retroactive bonuses based on that collaborative accountability system. Therefore, the six star facilities were truly the best in the state. I took over two no star facilities and turned them around by focusing the staff on attaining the six stars. Those providers who did not attain that status were incentivized to pursue each star and become the best. This system was thrown out by the corrupt Illinois Legislature because the big noncompliant owners did not want that accountability and distinction as a one or two star facility. This system works. The CMS five star obviously does not measure success only failure. An example of "Catch 23" that promises a star for every below average mistake rather than above average success then hangs those that make above average mistakes. (see Chapter 15 for more details on the failure of Monopsony incentives).

Gottcha with Catch 23

In the next chapters, it will be demonstrated how the monopsony restricts trade using catch 23 and controls enterprise to the point of being an oligarchy. The following are the tactics that the biggest bully enacts the monopsony to institutionalize American health care:

1. Government officials are immune from lawsuit.
2. Appeal rights that are decided by the perp and only adjudicated if the five levels of appeal can be financed at $500 per attorney hour for at least two thousand hours per issue before you can get to federal court, then it is another $2 million per case.
3. Licensing of all aspects of health care take away rights of due process.
4. Rules and regulations for controlling the operations discourage innovation.
5. Surveys of the licensees keep the victims in a state of fear of reprisal.
6. Civil money penalties and fines for noncompliance.
7. Enforcement proceedings can only accomplish fines, penalties, and jail time with no improvement in outcomes.
8. Appeal hearings administrated by government officials. Welcome to Kangaroo Court.
9. Building permits; no beds built in the last twenty-five years without approval of Big Brother. Where, oh, where is free enterprise?
10. Payment methods controlled by the Office of Budget and Finance.
11. Self-reporting of incidents (entrapment and self-incrimination).
12. Denial of claims without seeing the patient, and the money has been spent by the provider who cannot rebill the patient for any of it.
13. Hold on admissions because you did not comply with arbitrary and capricious rules.

14. Conditional license with revocation and if you admit we will cancel your license and kill your business.
15. Retaliation against providers. Don't talk back.
16. Patient rights with no provider rights. Consumer is always right, and the provider is always wrong and usually get sued.
17. Rule of law ignored by regulators. Why not most of them are attorneys?
18. Due process of law ignored by hearings offices and appeals process. Why not most of them are attorneys or offspring of attorneys or graduate liberals?

DUTY NO. 3—BIGGEST BULLY FAILURE

Health care is inductive in its quality standards/measures and the payment processes (paid on input units), not deductive (paid on outcome units measuring results):

- Hospitals are paid on DRGs, diagnosis-related groups (payment and quality incentives are paid on diagnoses, not outcome results).
- Physicians are paid on RVUs, relative value units (payment and quality measures are paid on treatment encounters, not on outcome results).
- Nursing homes are paid on RUGs, resource-utilization groups (payment and quality measures are paid on treatments, not on outcome results). If you get them better, your rate goes down.
- Home-care providers are paid on OASIS, outcome and assessment information set (payment and quality measures are paid on assessment, not on outcome results).
- Outpatient services are paid on OPPS, outpatient perspective payment system (payment and quality measures are paid on treatment, not on outcome results). Why would the biggest business in the world be paid differently than all other businesses who must provide a quality outcome to have income, while health care providers get paid whether they provide a quality product or service (referred to an outcome or a positive result) or not? Because the providers are happy not to be held responsible for results and the government wants to control the flow or resources so it does not have to prove a benefit, just a contribution to the cost . . . that they discount because the cost is too high. Providers do not want to be administratively accountable to outcome standards because they would have to define their products and services in relation to their costs per outcome unit, which they have never been required to do. Walah, the reason for escalating costs and deteriorating quality of life results.

Probably on the agenda of Congress, 99 percent of whom are golfers:

Affordable Golf Club Act—New Law: If you have old golf clubs, you can keep your golf clubs until April 2014. Author unknown but a visionary on our Congress!

The administration has passed a new law titled The Affordable Golf Club Act declaring that every citizen must purchase a new set of golf clubs before April 2014. This law has been passed, because until now, typically only the wealthy or financially responsible have been able to purchase new golf clubs without the assistance of their government. This new law ensures that every American can now have "affordable" golf clubs of their own, because everyone is equally entitled to new golf clubs. And if you want to keep the golf clubs you already have, you can do that until April 2014.

These affordable golf clubs will cost from $1,000 to $3,000 each depending on your income level. This does not include taxes, pull carts, electric-cart fees, greens fees, membership fees, balls, tees, gloves, range finders, storage fees, maintenance, or repair costs. In order to make sure everyone participates and purchases their affordable golf clubs, the costs of owning golf clubs will increase 50 percent each year up to 400 percent by year 2018. This way, wealthy people will pay more for something that other people don't want or can't afford to maintain. People who can't afford or refuse to maintain their golf clubs will be fined. However, children under the age of twenty-six can use their parents' golf clubs until they turn twenty-seven, at which time they must purchase their own golf clubs.

If you don't want or think you don't need golf clubs, you are still required to buy them. If you refuse to buy a set or make claims that you can't afford them, you will be fined $800 until you purchase a set or face imprisonment. People living in farming areas, ghettos, inner cities, Wyoming, or areas with no access to golf courses are not exempt. Age, health, prior experience or no experience are not acceptable excuses for not buying, maintaining, and using your golf clubs.

A government review board that doesn't know the difference between a hook and a slice will decide everything. This includes when, where, how often, and for what purposes you can use your golf clubs along with how many people can ride in your golf cart. The board will also determine if participants are too old or not healthy enough to be able to use their golf clubs. They will also decide if your golf clubs have outlived their usefulness or if you must purchase specific accessories, like a range finder with slope adjustment or a newer and more expensive set of golf clubs.

*Those that can afford memberships at expensive golf country clubs will be required to buy memberships. If you are already a member and you like your membership, you can keep your membership. After April 2014, a different country club will be assigned for you to purchase a membership.

Government officials are exempt from this new law as they and their families and some of their friends and a few of their friends can obtain golf clubs at the taxpayers' expense.

The Rule of Law

The **rule of law** (also known as nomocracy) is the **legal** principle that **law** should govern a nation, as opposed to arbitrary decisions by individual government officials.

Under the rule of law, the law is preeminent and can serve as a check against the abuse of power. Under rule by law, the law is a mere tool for a government that suppresses its power in a legalistic fashion.

Rule of law implies that every citizen is subject to the law, including law makers themselves. In this sense, it stands in contrast to an oligarchy, where the rulers are held above the law (which is not necessary by definition but which is typical). Lack of the rule of law can be found in democracies and dictatorships, and can happen because of neglect or ignorance of the law, or lack of corrective mechanisms for administrative abuse. Such as democracies with a rule-of-law culture, with a practice for redress of grievances, and fair hearing.

The functional interpretation of the term "rule of law", consistent with the traditional English meaning, contrasts the "rule of law" with the rule of man." According to the functional view, a society in which government officers have a great deal of discretion has a low degree of "rule of law", whereas a society in which government officers have little discretion has a high degree of "rule of law". Upholding the rule of law can sometimes require the punishment of those who commit offenses that are under but not statutory law. The rule of law is thus somewhat at odds with flexibility, even when flexibility may be preferable

The substantive interpretation holds that the rule of law intrinsically protects some or all individual rights by the restriction of the arbitrary exercise of power by subordinating it to well-defined established laws with enforcement in accordance with due process of law and its Fifth Amendment rights.

Why is the State of Iowa immune from following their own rules? The Department of Inspections and Appeals (DIA) violate due process in their conduct and allegations of noncompliance in a punitive and bullying manner.

The providers are held hostage by the surveyors for subjective interpretations of regulations, and punitive tactics are used that have destroyed the creativity and initiative of the providers, thereby creating fear factors used to blame the providers, causing a culture of incompetence that impedes the delivery of positive quality of life for the patients.

The doctrine of the rule of law dictates that government must be conducted according to law. Judges have identified three essential elements of the Constitution that were indicative of the rule of law:

1. Absence of due process before the law.
2. Equality Before the Law.
3. The Constitution is a result of the ordinary law of the land without prejudice.

The restriction of the arbitrary exercise of power by subordinating it to well define and established laws and enforcement procedures.

Administrative Procedures Act (each law passed by Congress and signed by the President has a statement regarding enforcement known as the Administrative Procedures for that bill pursuant to the Administrative Procedures Act APA Standard of Judicial Review)

Standard of Judicial Review

The APA requires that in order to set aside agency action not subject to formal trial-like procedures, the court must conclude that the regulation is "arbitrary and capricious, an abuse of discretion, or otherwise not in accordance with the law." However, Congress may further limit the scope of judicial review of agency actions by including such language in the organic statute. To set aside formal rule-making or formal adjudication whose procedures are trial-like (*see* APA, 5 U.S.C 556 standard of review allows courts to question agency action more strongly. For these more formal actions, agency decisions must be supported by "substantial evidence" after the court reads the "whole record," which can be thousands of pages long.

> Unlike arbitrary and capricious review, substantial evidence review gives the courts leeway to consider whether an agency's factual and policy determinations were warranted in light of all the information before the agency at the time of decision. Accordingly, arbitrary and capricious review is understood to be more deferential to agencies than substantial evidence review. Arbitrary and capricious review allows the agency's decisions to stand as long as an agency can give a reasonable explanation for its decision based on the information it had at the time. In contrast, the courts tend to look much harder at decisions resulting from trial-like procedures because those agency procedures resemble actual trial court procedures, but the Article III of the Constitution reserves the judicial powers for actual courts. Accordingly, courts are strict under the substantial evidence standard when agencies act like courts because being strict gives courts final say, preventing agencies from using too much judicial power, in violation of the doctrine of separation of powers.

The separation of powers doctrine is less of an issue with rule-making not subject to trial-like procedures. Such rule-making gives agencies a lot more leeway in court because it is much more like the legislative process reserved for Congress in Article II. The courts' main role here is ensuring that the agency rules line up with the Constitution and with the agency's statutory commands from Congress. Even if a court finds a rule very unwise, it will stand as long as it is not "arbitrary and capricious, an abuse of discretion, or otherwise not in accordance with the law."

Government Commits Fraud and Abuse

While government has the lawmakers creating immunity from the law due process for themselves and big government, which is required by the Fifth Amendment, it is being discarded for enforcement and civil money penalties without regard to appeals as mandated by the Administrative Procedure Act for every law enacted.

Parallel to Big Government

Adolph Hitler Quotes

"By the skillful and sustained use of propaganda, one can make a people see even heaven as hell or an extremely wretched life as paradise."

"How fortunate for governments that the people they administer don't think."

"Any alliance whose purpose is not the intention to wage war is senseless and useless."

"If you tell a big enough lie and tell it frequently enough, it will be believed."

Joseph Stalin Quotes

"When we hang the capitalists, they will sell us the rope."

"The death of one man is a tragedy. The death of millions is a statistic."

"Education is a weapon, whose effect depends on who holds it in his hands and at whom it is aimed."

"People who cast the votes decide nothing. The people who count the votes decide everything."

Racketeer Influenced and Corrupt Organizations Act

Racketeer Influenced and Corrupt Organizations Act, commonly referred to as the **RICO Act** or simply **RICO**, is criminal penalties for civil acts performed as a part of ongoing disregard for due process of law. The RICO Act focuses specifically on but has been used to indict government officials for intentionally circumventing the rule of law for their own purposes, as did Al Capone in his heyday.

- One of the most famous American gangsters, Al Capone, also known as "Scarface," rose to infamy as the leader of the Chicago mafia during the Prohibition era. Before being sent to Alcatraz Prison in 1931 from a tax evasion conviction, he had amassed a personal fortune estimated at $100 million and was responsible for countless murders.
- A crackdown on racketeering in Chicago meant that Al Capone's first mobster job was to move operations to Cicero. With the assistance of his brothers Frank (Salvatore) and Ralph, Capone infiltrated the government and police departments. Between them they took leading positions within Cicero city government in addition to running brothels, gambling clubs and racetracks.
- Capone kidnapped opponents' election workers and threatened voters with violence. He eventually won office in Cicero but not before his brother Frank had been killed in a shootout with Chicago's police force.

- Capone had prided himself on keeping his temper under wraps but when friend and fellow hood Jack Guzik was assaulted by a small-time thug, Capone tracked the assailant down and shot him dead in a bar. Due to lack of witnesses, Capone got away with the murder, but the publicity surrounding the case gave him a notoriety that he had never had before.

A prime example of RICO activity are the Obama Medicare cuts that are illegal, fraudulent, and abusive to patients and providers. The government agencies (who are immune from accountability for enforcement tactics) continue to accuse the private sector of fraud and abuse and have contracted with private consulting firms to dig up audit claims for Medicare overpayment that the auditors may deem to be abuse of the Medicare reimbursement system and fraud toward the beneficiaries. When these auditors ask for claims to review, they threaten the providers with denials first, recovery of past Medicare payments made, and take a no-prisoners approach. For this, the auditors are paid 25 percent of the dollars recovered even though the providers have five stages of appeal rights. Also, fraud in this vein does not require intent on the part of the provider be proven, only the opinion of the RAC auditors is needed to trigger a fraud charge, potential jail time, and a possible five-year exclusion from practicing in a Medicare provider business.

First of all, the Medicare trust funds are not the government's money. It belongs to the beneficiaries who have paid in the money. Secondly, the government has been depriving the elderly their Medicare benefits using denial of payment and the RAC (recovery audit contractor) audit gestapo tactics to suppress Medicare coverage for beneficiaries. This is while the Medicare trust-fund money was loaned to the general fund for fighting the Iraq and Afghanistan wars to the tune of $700 billion. All that is left in the fund are US Treasury Bills while Congress claims that entitlements to Medicare are our biggest problem from a budgetary standpoint. Wrong! Big government fraud is our biggest problem.

Without government involvement, the Medicare program has a surplus and takes in 40 percent more than it pays out for health-care claims. Even with the paying agent CMS (Centers of Medicare and Medicaid Services) depriving the elderly their benefits using fear tactics against the providers, Medicare pays its bills timely if they meet stringent interpretive guidelines, while Medicaid goes further into the Obama Care hole. Since 1975 when HEW, the Federal Department of Health Education and Welfare, started denying Medicare claims as not being medically necessary or not improving the patients' functioning, some thirty million seniors over sixty-five years of age have been deprived of their full entitled one-hundred-day-per-spell-of-illness skilled-nursing benefit due to the imposition of a little-known rule that allowed the government to review claims and retrospectively take money back. This started the suppression of Medicare Part A and B benefits for the elderly to the tune of $600 billion since 1975 to the present and the elderly's purportedly beneficiaries' right to be restored *to their highest level of functioning* and discharged back to the community.

As the denials rose to almost 50 percent of the submitted claims in the 1980s and '90s, the providers started to cut back on the provided days of Medicare Part A skilled care, and as a result, more patients were having their long-term care paid by Medicaid that by law is not to be billed until the Medicare benefits are exhausted. Then to make things worse, the government changed the retrospective review and recovery to prospective denial of payment even though the provider in good faith had provided the care and paid for medications, therapy treatments, medical supplies, and medical equipment. This further cut back on the amount of days the providers were willing to risk to the whims of the government claims; reviewers, who were just looking at documents, weren't even medical professionals, and medical necessity had not been reviewed by a qualified physician. This is fraud at its worst as the government literally ignored the patient's need and the provider's loss under the guise the claims were not medically necessary or did not improve the patients' condition. The truth was, the bureaucrats did not want to pay and exceeded the inadequate budget constraints.

To support this allegation of fraud and abuse by the federal government, there are two federal court cases that convicted them of this fact for which they have ignored and continued to flaunt:

Fox v. Bowen, Connecticut 1986

In 1986, a Connecticut Federal Judge in a lawsuit (*Fox v. Bowen*) determined HCFA (now CMS) had violated Medicare beneficiaries' entitled constitutional rights to skilled-nursing services and ordered HCFA to revise the skilled-nursing manual to clarify the requirements for coverage under Medicare Part A. The court ordered them to reopen fourteen thousand cases and pay for the skilled care. The court also ordered HCFA to look for a "reason to pay" instead of a "reason not to pay." The court's purpose was to ensure Medicare claims are approved when the requirements for skilled care (licensed nursing, licensed therapists, and licensed social workers) are met.

Transmittal 262

As a result of *Fox v. Bowen*, HCFA took action in 1987 by issuing Transmittal 262 but never sent this information to the providers. It was only sent to the fiscal intermediaries who offered no education or training on the transmittal or the court-ordered process, nor have they placed the order in practice during the past twenty-six years. As a result the one-hundred-day stay was cut down to an average length of stay (ALOS) of twenty-two days and, during the 1990s, began to rise to an ALOS of thirty-four days. With the initiation of the RAC audits, the purge is starting again to deprive the patients of their rightful Medicare-entitled health-care benefits in skilled-nursing facilities.

Jimmo v. Sibelius, Vermont 2012

One of the tactics that has been used by CMS was to deny Medicare Part A skilled claims if the skilled patient "reached their prior level of functioning." This was subjective, as at what point do you look for their prior level of functioning, but more importantly, as stated by the court ruling, "neither the Medicare statute nor the implementing regulations refer to or suggest an improvement standard." The federal court again has ordered CMS to reissue its interpretive guidelines, its manuals, its operating policies and pay retroactively only back to January 2011 based on claims filed and denied. This, of course, will not pay for the $600 billion fraud committed over the years due to the misapplication and misinterpretation of the Medicare laws and regulations on the Medicare beneficiaries. This also does not touch the amount of the fraud the government has caused due to most providers not even submitting claims in fear of denial and possible fraud allegations. The true amount of potentially applicable underpayments by the government (CMS) cannot be proven as a result of Medicare claims not being filed due to fear tactics conducted by the government. The government cannot be sued unless a Medicare claim has been submitted and denied. Effectively, the government knowingly underpaid and denied Medicare claims but also never will pay the unfiled Medicare claims just mentioned above. Medicare beneficiaries should be vehemently upset due to not receiving their rightful Medicare entitlements! Additional government settlements will not be paid unless there is a class action of providers who have had Medicare beneficiaries denied claims. Until claimants join the class action lawsuit together, this governmental fraud is going to continue.

Obama Care and other politicians further this fraud and abuse of the elderly and disabled by stating they will be cutting Medicare funding—or will propose further cuts to Medicare.

States, many of whom are facing budgetary woes, have also been affected through the misapplication of Medicare laws, rules, and regulations as Medicaid is to be the payer of last resort, meaning if someone has Medicare and meets the requirements for skilled care, Medicare should have paid before the States' Medicaid programs were subjected to fraudulent costs to cover the resulting long-term care. Again, I reiterate, the money does not belong to Congress, the president, or the Supreme Court—it belongs to you and me as we have it withheld from our wages throughout our entire working careers.

It is time Americans became educated and involved in how their money is wasted and turned against American businesses by government. Government-paid auditors (more realistically should be classified as bounty hunters) have only one thing in mind. Twenty-five percent of billions, potentially trillions and zillions of recovered provider income is a lot of contingency fees—even though it is disguised as provider fraud and abuse.

THE CURRENT VA DEBACLE IS AN EXAMPLE OF MONOPSONY (GOVERNMENT) RUN HEALTH CARE

Why would the VA Hospitals not contract with skilled nursing facilities that have upwards to 200,000 empty beds nationally? Veterans predominately need long term rehabilitation and restorative services not just Government run acute care.

Why would I bring this up? My wife, son and I own two skilled nursing homes that have applied for a contract with VA and have been prevented from getting the opportunity to help solve the wait time problem because we are not a 3 to 5 star provider using the Government's flawed performance rating and cannot meet their arbitrary financial stability standards; sounds systemic doesn't it?

We have a 100 beds in Muscatine, Iowa with 15 available for vets and in Washington we have 125 beds with 75 available for vets to assist in providing much needed restorative care for the returning veterans. Why wouldn't the use of the private sector to solve the problem of wait times and getting veterans back home work? It would if the bureaucrats would get out of the way. We have 4 vets at the present time, utilizing the Medicaid program rather than VA benefits. This shifts Federal costs inappropriately to the State of Iowa Medicaid costs.

In Muscatine All-American Care has restored and returned 260 patients back into the community. We offer full therapy, skilled nursing, post-acute care, pre acute care together with psychosocial groups, clubs and classes with the mission of returning 57% of our admissions back out of dependent health care principally now being paid for by Medicaid. We utilize the Medicare benefits as required by law for up to 100 days of restorative care so the patients can return to their real homes. We have served up to 10 vets, at a time, utilizing the Medicaid program for the last two and one half years rather than VA benefits. This shifts Federal costs inappropriately to the State of Iowa Medicaid costs.

So, yes we are not three stars and have filed for Chapter 11 protection due to the sanctions imposed on our Washington facility for minor violations. We have been prevented from admitting patients seven of the twenty –six months we have owned the facility and fined $100,000 since we purchased this dump that was allowed to stay in compliance for years because the owner was politically connected. Not only have we been subjected to illegal arbitrary and capricious tactics by Rod Roberts (who has never set foot in our facilities) and his Gestapo crew but cannot assist the VA hospitals in the area to shorten wait times and restore veterans back into the community. Rather we have lost over $1 million dollars because of Government run health care.

We have been black listed by the State as one of the worst facilities in the Iowa due to our political views. The Des Moines Register's self-appointed watchdog Clark Kaufman is allowed to distort and defame independently owned nursing homes, such as ours, without proof based on what the State's arbitrary and capricious surveys publish on the internet without due process of law ... true or not. We have invited him to visit our facilities that he continues to incriminate and distort without investigating the facts.

Our facilities are extraordinarily clean, odor free and have more than the average nursing homes RNs, LPNs, CNAs, Therapists, social workers, rehab aides and have had $1 million dollars in renovation and successfully changed the culture of staff from not caring to being committed to the restoration of our patients. Thus making our facilities into a home like environment; and an effective private enterprise to innovate and improve the care of the disabled and elderly veterans so they can go back home.

It is our opinion that Obama Monopsony Care will only exacerbate these budgetary glitches and service blunders. God save the American Enterprise system from Government control. Let the creators create and the politicians debate.

PART II
CATCH 23

CHAPTER ONE

CATCH 23

The Law Took a Bite Out of Me

It said
I was to agree
With the decree
Regardless of the fee

My attorney
Asserted he was not free
Forcing my business
To a take a knee
Or get a law degree

What I said happened
To enterprise
That is surmised
To be free
In the country "'tis of thee"

Uncle Sam threw the book at me
Catch me if you can
As I file for bankruptcy
On the perpetrator's stand

Taking the fifth
To avoid catch 23
Before it buries me

Then the judicious bully
Put me in the loser's jail
Because I fail

To commit perjury

Under catch 23

MONOPSONY DISREGARDS THE RULE OF LAW

The lawmakers make themselves immune from due process of laws they create to immune themselves from such accountability and prevent the abused to get justice. The governed are enabled to appeal at any time, but it is too expensive for the victims of monopsony to appeal, creating catch 23.

> In the Land of Oz
> The people do as Oz does
> As Oz is
> And as Oz wants
> But the fact is
> Oz never was
> And never
> Will be
> For you or me

Government Corruption
The Bleeping Giant in the Land of OZ

Can a corrupt government be stopped? Yes, but first, the people have to recognize the corruption and be committed to eradicate it. Following is an example of the impact of government over reaching and becoming the perpetrator of corruption.

Nursing homes have been the bane of society ever since the first well-meaning nurse decided to take care of the declining elderly in a home-like environment. During the 1940s, due to the pressures of war and the return of the soldiers, these rest homes began to crop up as a way to congregate nursing care and relieve the immediate family of the responsibility so they could get on with their jobs and child bearing.

Now sixty-some years later, the nursing home is considered the last place a person wants to go. Why would a well-intended beginning have such an unfortunate ending? What? I thought we still need nursing homes. Not if government has its way. The use or misuse of power is the reason. It is now health care, not the venue of the real estate magnets that typically own them. So we are going to put them out of business because they do not comply with the bureaucrats' version of end-of-life care.

The travesty is, the large chain operators of nursing homes are given a pass when it comes to enforcement. The rules are enforced on the mom-and-pops to force them into the conglomerate's hands because, of course, the big businesses are the only ones that are cost conscious and efficient in their misuse of the taxpayers' money. CMS, the Centers of Medicare and Medicaid, as the enforcement arm of the Department of Health and Human Services lords over those that do not have the resources to fight back when the rules become the tools of "do it or die" tactics. It is all subject to their interpretation and prejudicial rule.

Now we come to the reason for this article. It is the diabolical result of this situation that is driving us toward socialized decisions by government to pigeonhole the elderly into "end of life" death panels under the guise of cost containment and reversal of entitlements that are not entitlements at all. The Medicare program is not an entitlement; it is the individual's own money. It is entrusted to government to collect, preserve, and distribute the funds as each individual needs the care in a hospital, nursing home, or at home. Not only has the money been misappropriated but borrowed by the general fund to fight wars and set up an enforcement system that makes the gestapo look tame.

How is this possible without outrage by the baby boomers, the AARP members, the political parties, the watchdog groups, etc.? Because it is done with treasuries that are sold to the Medicare trust funds so the pirates can utilize the elderly's money without them knowing it then blame the so-called entitlements for our economic problems. For more than fifty years, this government corruption has been perpetrated upon the Medicare beneficiaries to hide the fact that the intent of the Medicare law is to restore the elderly back to their homes using holistic methods during the one-hundred-day recuperative period for each spell of illness. This insurance policy that we all pay for has never changed since being enacted into law in 1964 as part of the Great Society programs.

What, I thought Medicare is ever changing for the betterment of society? Well, that is what CMS and the Congress want us to think. They want to control the funding and utilize the money for their budgetary games. How would I know this? Well, I was around in 1965 when Medicare was being rolled out by Blue Cross of America under contract as the first fiscal intermediary for processing the claims. I worked for Arthur Andersen & Co., who had a contract with Hospital Corporation of America to assist Blue Cross in the implementation of the billing and cost-reporting procedures required by the newly released Hospital and Nursing Home regulations. I was told by my superiors at AA&Co. that I was to be an expert in this endeavor and have been involved in it ever since.

From my vantage point, the following has transpired over the years into the government corruption we have today. The prime example of the misuse of the Medicare funding was the required one-hundred-day stay in a nursing home if the patient had a three-day stay in a hospital. In those days, it was not unusual for an elderly patient to reside in the hospital for twenty-five days recuperating from multiple diagnoses. So the Congress rule writers established the benefit period to be one hundred days per spell of illness (defined as medical necessity, followed by severity of the illness, resulting in interventions by licensed professionals for restoring the patient to their highest level of functioning so they could return home). If the patient was able to return to functioning enough to enable them to be free of hospital or nursing-home care for sixty days and needed another three-day stay in the hospital, they would qualify for another one-hundred-day recuperative period.

Here is where the corruption began. CMS, then termed HEW (Department of Health, Education, and Welfare), decided to misinterpret the one-hundred-day stay as their right to interpret medical necessity using arbitrary and capricious terms to deny claims submitted by the nursing homes. The skilled-nursing facilities (SNF) had to be certified by HEW to qualify for providing and billing for the services. In good faith, they would provide the care and incur the therapy and medication costs as well as the expensive labor costs for nurses, therapists, and social workers and the government fiscal intermediary. In those days, Aetna Insurance Company would deny the claim and take back the money. The reasoning being Aetna's interpretation that the patient did not improve enough to qualify or the documentation was not good enough or the results were not enough to warrant reimbursement.

In those days, HEW was trying to reduce the one-hundred-day benefit to the first twenty days before the coinsurance period of eighty days kicked in. This way, the patient had to be discharged from Medicare so they did not have to share in the next eighty days even if they needed it to get well. Then the patient either had to go home too soon or stay in the SNF spending down their own assets at an exorbitant rate to qualify for the true entitlement program, Medicaid. Over the years, some thirty million elderly patients have been deprived of their rightful extended caré benefits because of this denial process. The nursing homes then began to ramp down their restorative programming to just the therapies and deny any other services such as skilled nursing and discharge planning because HEW was denying the claims.

Of course, the rule makers put in the right to appeal these aberrant denials under a catch 23 ruling that the provider could appeal back to Aetna, who had denied the claim in the first place, and get another denial and then proceed through four more levels of government appeals if they want to incur the costs of attorneys and accountants, then lose anyway. This tactic, of course, reduced the incidence of Medicare claims for SNFs by 75 percent, and the elderly were relegated most times to an end-of-life sentence on Medicaid, the true entitlement that has now become the resting place for all of the Obama Care recipients. Ironically, the tactic was to have saved the government billions when, in fact, it is costing their fiscal future in trillions, not billions.

(Ironically, hospitals can turn away the indigent while nursing homes cannot. Hospitals now can garnish wages for nonpayment; nursing homes cannot. Hospitals can discharge for nonpayment; nursing homes cannot. Hospitals are paid for illness; nursing homes are paid less for wellness.)

Why then did the government get away with this corruption? Well, they didn't. In 1984, Grandma Fox's grandson sued HEW (*Fox v. Bowen*) for depriving his grandmother therapy benefits in a skilled-nursing facility, and the judge found in their favor two years later and ordered the HEW to rewrite their interpretative guidelines for coverage. The judge decided that HEW was depriving the patients in SNFs their constitutional right to due process and was depriving them of the benefit they had paid for. Some $350 million in claims were reopened and paid. The judge ordered HEW to release new and broader interpretive guidelines under Release 262 and educate the providers on the fact that the government was not to deny coverage because of arbitrary and capricious words such as "not improving because of reaching a plateau" and "not having restorative potential."

Release 262 was buried by HEW, and Aetna never did educate the providers on the rights of the beneficiaries when, in fact, HEW changed the way they paid Aetna from number of claims paid to number of claims denied, and the denial rates reached 50 percent in the 1980s, and the average length of coverage was driven down to twenty-two from one hundred, and more patients were relegated to an end-of-life sentence on Medicaid. This government corruption has cost the taxpayer a trillion dollars in waste over the thirty years and continues to be the tactic of CMS: intimidation through enforcement tactics threatening providers with fraud and abuse charges if they extend the coverages to one hundred days. CMS was then sued again by the Medicare Center for advocacy in the *Jimmo v. Sibelius* case, losing again for using the term "must improve" to qualify for Medicare coverage, thus depriving the beneficiaries their right to Medicare coverage for illnesses resulting in a three-day hospital stay.

But again, CMS dodges the corruption bullet by allowing hospitals to avoid the three-day hospital stay using the term "observation day" even though the patient is in the hospital and is receiving hospital care just to further deprive the beneficiaries who have paid for the insurance and deprive society and its burgeoning baby boomers their health care.

Now for my story and how it impacts those that know the situation and have tried to make corrections and changes that will solve the problems of funding and care of the elderly who are thwarted and abused by the federal and state government without compunction. Over the last fifty years, I have been involved in servicing and educating hospitals, nursing homes, home health care, assisted living, and physicians on the Medicare rules and regulations stemming from the laws passed in 1964 and 1965. After leaving Arthur Andersen in 1968, I became a partner in two CPA firms, heading up their health-care practices and advising them on the rules and regulations pertaining to Medicare and Medicaid. I became the nursing-home associations both state and national reimbursement consultant for negotiating with government how to set rates and hold the providers accountable.

This is where the story gets complicated. The government at all levels does not allow for challenging their interpretations and actions without repercussions. In my case, my accounting and consulting businesses were founded on challenging the denial of payment to SNFs due to arbitrary and capricious reasons that the federal courts had found them guilty of doing. We successfully were able to assist over 140 skilled-nursing facilities to bill and collect over one hundred thousand claims resulting in forty thousand more elderly being restored and returned home. If the government denied the claims, we appealed and won them all because of our documentation and knowledge of what the federal courts had decided until the Administrative Law Judges were moved from the Social Security Administration to CMS and now just rubber-stamp everything the corruption machine enacts.

In 2009, my wife, son, and I decided to exit the consulting business because the depression of 2007 forced the nursing homes into a cutback mode and our business was cut in half. So we purchased a skilled-nursing facility in Muscatine, Iowa. That's when CMS and the State of Iowa bureaucrats began retaliating against our views and service procedures. Following is that gory story:

RAMIFICATIONS OF STATE OF IOWA DEPARTMENT OF INSPECTIONS AND APPEALS PUNITIVE ACTIONS—ALL-AMERICAN RESTORATIVE CARE OF WASHINGTON

1. Jerry, Shari, and Kip Rhoads purchased the Washington 125 bed nursing home on October 11, 2011, three months after Governor Branstad toured their Muscatine facility and two months after Jerry Rhoads met with Rod Roberts, director of the Iowa Department of Inspections and Appeals, to propose collaborative surveys and change in payment system to pay for performance versus an average minimum per diem. Then the retaliation began in Washington.
2. December 23, 2011. There was an incident where a patient was lying on the floor for forty-eight minutes, fines of $20,000, hold on admissions for three months, published on the Internet and in the Des Moines *Register* before our appeals were adjudicated. We never recovered from this exaggerated incident. Patient who fell out of the sight of staff had a small bump on her head and was discharged to the psych unit afterward because of her behaviors that included habitually lying on the floor as a coping habit (she is bipolar and was previously homeless and slept under a bridge). Staff was alleged to not have intervened during the forty-eight minutes, but testimony by staff contradicted those allegations, but they were ignored due to lack of documentation. An amount of $65,000 in legal fees was incurred fighting the allegations, which are still being appealed. From that point forward, we were targeted by DIA for punishment and an example of their gestapo tactics to keep the other smaller providers in the fear mode.
3. February 7, 2012. Complaint survey, family member, regarding heat and staff sleeping.
4. February 28, 2012. Three G violations for the floor incident, $18,000 CMS fines, $2000 state fines, special-focus

designation with a hold on admissions by Rob Reck, who expanded the survey into falls, and the video allegation that is still in appeal two years later.

5. March 15, 2012. Complaint survey, family member.
6. April 9, 2012. Complaint survey—former employees.
7. April 12, 2012. Complaint survey.
8. April 25, 2012. Hold by CMS.
9. May 9, 2012. Revisit.
10. May 17, 2012. Annual survey.
11. June 13, 2012. Revisit.
12. July 3, 2012. Revisit.
13. September 25, 2012. Revisit passed; CMS hold lifted.
14. November 2. Complaint survey.
15. November 21, 2012. SNF biannual survey.
16. December 12, 2012. Revisit.
17. February 18, 2013. Complaint survey.
18. February. Steve Warneke, administrator.
19. March. Self-reported fall, $5,000 fines.
20. April 12, 2013. Plan of correction approved.
21. April 14, 2013. Failure to pass revisit; conditional license issued.
22. April 18, 2013. Revisit.
23. April 24, 2013. Hold on admissions. Alleged wound problem. Allegen State's consultant found no wound problems.
24. July 3, 2013. Revisit. Passed all twenty-three tags with no violations.
25. July 2013. Conditional license lifted.
26. June 2, 2013. Richard T. expired and received no CPR.
27. October 3, 2013. Complaint survey regarding kitchen, patient no. 1, and patient no. 2 by fired staff members.
28. November 7, 2013. Extended survey, immediate jeopardy for patient abuse of no. 2.
29. November 7, 2013. Conditional license imposed with $30,000 state fines; $48,000 CMS fines for immediate jeopardy (IJ) that is being appealed.
30. December. Complaint survey, revisit, six month survey, one tag for documentation of intake of fluids. December came of the fourth hold.

31. January 2014 received 2567 with two picky violations, but having a D severity keeps facility on conditional license, admission hold, and special focus furthering the retaliation against the owners.
32. Fire Marshall had a plan of correction that was not timely, and CMS put another admission hold on to be effective April 9, and the violations were cleared by April 1, but the hold was extended in error until August of 2014, so we got no Medicare money until the government screw up was reversed, and WPS had to pay $128,000 being wrongfully withheld with no interest of course.
33. Had a six month survey and annual in June with only five tags, and July 25, 2014, came off special focus.

Summary

From December 23, 2011, two months and twelve days after we took over a very noncompliant facility, we have had thirty-three visits or interventions by DIA and/CMS; 4,999 copies of records and pages of interviews with staff, former staff, families, patients; three IDR hearings; one ALJ hearing; one meeting in Des Moines with DHS, CMS, DIA; and a telephone call from CMS threatening closure. No patient was injured other than a bump on the head for the floor incident and one broken hip due to a fall; no significant wounds were found by the State's consultant, and for this, we were punished to the following extent:

- $104,000 in fines
- $70,000 in legal fees
- $1.4 million lost revenue due to the two admission holds and two conditional license allowing no admissions
- $128,000 in claims not paid for six months
- Defamation of Kip Rhoads by publishing an allegation regarding sexual contact with a delusional patient without investigating the fabricated incident that put Kip in the hospital with high blood pressure
- Defamation of the Rhoads family by the Des Moines *Register* and local news media without due process of law

- The bookkeeper and the dietary manager were selling food and taking the money. The bookkeeper feigned suicide in front of Kip Rhoads after the dietary manager was fired and Shari Rhoads was pressuring the bookkeeper to explain shortages in petty cash. The bookkeeper was actively looking for other employment after the dietary manager was fired then never showed up again after being hospitalized with the so-called suicide attempt.
- Census rose to sixty from forty-seven with no Medicare program in place to sixty, with twelve on Medicare by February survey hold that bottomed out at forty in mid-2012 and rose back up to fifty-four mid-2013 and is now back down to forty due to the nine months of admission holds imposed in the two years and three months we have owned the Washington facility, causing a loss of $1.4 million in revenue, creating $726,000 in operating losses in 2012 and $174,000 operating losses in 2013. Due to the $1 million financial borrowing that it took to keep the doors open, we have been forced to file chapter 11 bankruptcy for both the Washington operation and the Muscatine facility. The Rhoadses are being forced to sell both facilities as a result of the punitive actions by the State of Iowa Department of Inspections and Appeals (DIA) in retaliation for appeals and disagreements with the governor and the director of DIA.

Following is the condition of the noncompliant facility when we purchased it and what we invested immediately to modernize a dump and save the patients ... in other words we were there to save it:

1. 162 fluorescent bulbs burnt out and not replaced—$3,200
2. Eighty-four ballasts not replaced—$500
3. Carpeting dirty with urine odors—$2,660 to clean
4. No intercom system and old telephone system—$17,448
5. Old, antiquated beds and furniture—$31,000
6. Ugly curtains rather than blinds to let light in—new blinds, bedspreads, privacy curtains, $27,000
7. Dead trees in front—removal $2,332
8. Old signage and lighting system out front—$6,056

9. Flooding parking lot—sewer system had to be rerouted, $16,919
10. Parking lot with pot holes everywhere—new parking lot was necessary, $62,332
11. Roof leaked—new roof was necessary, $86,000
12. New gutters and down spouts—$9,750
13. Ugly, dirty red brick building—painted white, $13,000
14. No Internet, wireless computer systems—network and twenty work stations set up, $7,000
15. Clinical documentation system implemented—$6,750
16. Financial documentation system implemented—$10,000
17. Camera security system installed—$3,350
18. Medications documented manually—medications computerized, $10,000
19. Charting system was old and a mess—new charting system put in place, $5,350
20. Medical records was a series of unmarked boxes—medical records system put in place with new staff, $3,000
21. Old washers and dryers—new equipment leased, $7,000
22. Dietary kitchen disorganized, inefficient, and poor food—upgraded everything, including staff, $20,000
23. Old water heaters that had to be replaced—$16,000
24. Shower rooms were old and dirty—remodeled with new shower chairs, $10,000
25. Hospitality carts were old and dirty—replaced, $2,000
26. Patient rooms, doors, handrails, and floors were old and had odors—painted the rooms, handrails, and doors and cleaned all floors to get rid of odors, $27,000
27. Front patio replaced—$5,165
28. Building columns, lights, and flag poles installed—$5,150
29. Therapy equipment had to be purchased—$20,000
30. Renovation of the all-purpose room—$26,034
31. Entertainment center—$3,241
32. Total invested in renovations, systems, replacements, linens, inventory of food and supplies = $740,000, total secured bank debt $2.1 million

Everyone is asking, how does this happen? This noncompliant dump the Rhoadses purchased and made respectable was allowed to stay open while the regulators have made it impossible for the Rhoadses to stay in business. Also, how can you run a business when you cannot generate sales for seven months and have to deal with twenty-six interventions by the surveyors and 4,999 pages of documentation that have to be copied and provided the regulators to use against you.

Statements were taken from the patients and their families who had lived in the terrible conditions before the Rhoadss took over … "they wonder where the surveyors were when the former owner did nothing to make things better, but still passed them in their surveys".

RIPPLE AFFECT OF PUNITIVE ACTION BY DIA

1. Financial hardship imposed by DIA and CMS by fines, holds on admissions, prevention of referrals, defamation of reputation when published on the Internet and in the media before appeals, resulting in bankruptcy filings.
2. Employee morale is impacted and fear factor imposed by the regulators because of bullying tactics, phone calls, and civil money penalties.
3. Staff leaving because of fear of job security and possible holding of paychecks.
4. Staff recruiting and hiring impacted due to rumors and fear of further retaliation causing the facilities to close and not honor paychecks.
5. Patients and families expressing concern and threats if facilities are forced to close because of enforcement tactics and fines.
6. Communities are concerned about losing 160 jobs and the availability of long-term care beds.
7. Ownership's financial future put in serious jeopardy with no recourse for holding the agencies accountable for arbitrary and capricious tactics used to retaliate against the providers.
8. Self-reporting of incidents is in affect entrapment and not legal.
9. Interviewing terminated employees to dig up incriminating, distorted information used to bully the owners.
10. Employee interviews are used against the owners by slanting the questions and intimidation of the staff and patients.

11. Informal dispute resolution is not objective and does not follow the Administrative Procedure Act.
12. On-site surveyors are mean-spirited, arbitrary, and subjective in their investigation using illegal tactics for digging up allegations then distorting them in long-winded 2567 reports leading to exaggerated severity codes and resulting fines.

For more complete details on proposed solutions to the Monopsony enforcement procedures, I have written several books on the topics of reinforcement and quality of life incentives versus fines, penalties and intimidation:

1. *Eldercide, You Don't Know What You Don't Know*, iUniverse 2009
2. *Restore Elder Pride, Shift The Paradigm*, iUniverse 2012
3. *The Boomers Are Coming*, Xlibris 2013
4. *American in the Red Zone*, Xlibris 2013
5. *Never Too Old to Live*, Xlibris 2012
6. *Cost Accounting for Long Term Care*, American Health Care Association 1981/2000
7. *How to Win the Monopsony Game*, Caregiver Management Systems, 2000
8. *Biggest Bully in the China Closet*, All-American Care, 2014

CHAPTER TWO

WILL MONOPSONY CARE FIX HEALTH-CARE PROBLEMS?

An e-mail letter to Jerry Rhoads from the future president of the United States—

Senator Barack Obama

Dear Jerry:

Thank you for taking the time to contact me. I apologize for the delay in my response. Quite frankly, I was unprepared for the volume of correspondence and e-mails I have received since coming to the Senate in January, 2005 and I am just now finally feeling more comfortable about my ability to respond in a timely manner to the thousands of communications I receive each week from Illinois residents. Your particular comments about what I should be doing in Washington to improve access to needed health care are greatly appreciated.

Thank you for sharing the ecaregiver.com model of care with me. As it states, we must use methodology and systems that allow health care providers to more accurately assess patient needs, provide high quality care, hold health care professionals responsible for outcomes, and create a culture of patient safety.

Be certain that improving and strengthening our nation's health care system is a priority of mine. Thank you for contributing to the debate surrounding this call for improvement.

There should be no question that the President's proposed cuts in Medicare and Medicaid will result in the denial of needed care. To me, these cuts, in a budget that extends the President's tax cuts, reflect a distorted sense of national priorities, and I will fight them.

Sincerely,

Barack Obama

United States Senator

Commentaries by Jerry Rhoads, Author

After passing the Affordable Health Care Act of 2010, the Obama administration offered the states new ways to improve care, lower costs for Medicaid by *improving care quality for nursing facility residents* (however, at a cost of $1 trillion for demonstration projects and another $1trillion in enforcement of new regulations over the next ten years, healthcare administration costs will double)(To date the private insurance premiums have increased 84% in Iowa, leading the States with 49% nationwide, to pass through the unaffordable costs of Obama Care).

In 1971 when Nixon Administration instituted wage and price controls for businesses including hospitals I was a partner in an accounting firm that got the assignment of auditing requested price increases by Catholic Hospitals. We were to examine their records and determine if their request for a price increase was supported by the related costs. This was first time hospitals had been required to relate costs to specific procedures not just total average costs per inpatient day. We discovered that there were no cost accounting systems in place to track costs by diagnosis, treatment, test or by discharge or by outcome. As a result the project fell on the integrity of the hospital's management to justify their escalating prices to the insurance companies.

Now in 2014 under the Affordable Patient Care Act they are being asked to produce the same records to justify their escalating prices and the story is the same ... we don't have systems in place to cost specific services. But now their integrity is being challenged and will result in only certain health plans putting them in their network. If they aren't in the network and they admit a patient out of network the patient will get stuck with the sizable bill ... and now hospitals have the authority to garnish their future. So the Affordable Act has created another monster called bankruptcies it was to have prevented. It will do just the opposite—make it more complicated for the practitioner without any improvement in results. That is the history of government- and State-run hospitals and the VA health system failure.

The Centers of Medicare/Medicaid Services announced today a new initiative to help states improve the quality of care for people in nursing homes. Nearly two-thirds of nursing facility residents are receiving Medicaid benefits, and most are also eligible for Medicare benefits. The CMS Innovation Center in collaboration with the CMS Medicare-Medicaid Coordination Office will establish a new demonstration focused on reducing preventable inpatient hospitalizations among residents of nursing facilities by providing these individuals with the treatment they need without having to unnecessarily go to a hospital. Hospitalizations are often expensive, disruptive, disorienting, and dangerous for frail elders and people with disabilities and cost Medicare billions of dollars each year. CMS-funded research on Medicare-Medicaid eligible nursing facility residents in 2005 found that almost 40 percent of hospital admissions were preventable, accounting for 314,000 potentially avoidable hospitalizations and $2.6 billion in Medicare expenditures.

Starting in the fall of 2011, CMS will competitively select independent accountable care organizations (ACOs) to partner with and implement evidence-based interventions at interested nursing facilities. These interventions could include using nurse practitioners in nursing facilities, supporting transitions between hospitals and nursing facilities, and implementing best practices to prevent falls, pressure ulcers, urinary tract infections, or other events that lead to poor health outcomes and expensive hospitalizations. Additionally, this initiative supports the administration's Partnership for Patients goal of reducing hospital readmission rates by 20 percent by the end of 2013.

COMMENTARY

ACOs are a brainchild of university demonstration projects and enforcement thereof: universities and think tanks, which have never operated a health-care business, be it a hospital, nursing home, or medical practice, are employed by CMS to tell them what they already have decided—keep it administratively simple but complex enough to be ineffective so as to control the flow of dollars to certain providers to keep them quiet. Enforcement is to create the aura of the bad guys in private business, ripping off the poor to become rich, when the effect it will have is that the poor and aging Americans will be left out in the cold as the dollars are rationed to the younger population. Enforcement will increase the size of the government agency and build on fear as a deterrent. So goes health reform—no real initiatives to move from an illness-based payment system to a wellness-based payment for outcomes, not incomes.

COMMENTARY

> This 2,500-page giant piece of social legislation is nothing other than a political tactic to keep control over $3 trillion of American taxpayers' money. It throws the private sector under the truck full of perks for universities and think tanks using grants and consulting contracts, resulting in more social regulations dictated by the federal government, leading us to believe that the vast health care legislation protects us from the horrible insurance companies, the greedy providers, and the ignorance of voters.
>
> In reality, it is one thing to repeal health care reform and another to reform the wasteful spending going on. We pay for illness, not wellness; we pay for pills, not stronger wills; and we pay for incomes, not outcomes. Until we take the authority for determining how to pay away from the bureaucrats, insurance companies, and academics, we will continue to bankrupt the current Medicare, Medicaid, and insurance plans.

AFFORDABLE—NOT

PATIENT PROTECTION AND AFFORDABLE CARE ACT
(i.e., Obama Care)

Affordable—Not . . .
Protecting the elderly and disabled—Not

Projected Cost =

$465 Billion for State Exchanges
$434 Billion Medicaid Increases
$176 Billion Demonstration Projects and Enforcement
$1.075 Trillion Annul Cost

Projected Funding =

$414 Billion Medicare Cuts
$349 Billion Provider Taxes
$210 Billion Medicare Withholding Taxes and Surtaxes
$107 Billion Pharmacy, Hospital Taxes
$ 68 Billion Fines and Penalties
$150 Billion Cadillac Insurance Taxes
$ 13 Billion Downsizing Medical Savings Accounts
$ 20 Billion Taxes on Devices
$ 15 Billion Reductions in Tax Deduction for Medical Expenses
$ 3 Billion Taxes on Tanning Salons
$1.218 Trillion Annual Taxes and Reductions in Benefits

So President Obama who said it won't cost taxpayers one dime was either lying or overzealous in his sales job. Now we are being told by Professor Gruber the economist who designed the system for him that they lied to get it passed. And if it had been know about the above cost and funding debacle it would have never gotten by the so called ignorant consumers. And it was sold on macroeconomics assuming that the economy was going to turn around and income taxes would be sufficient to overcome the shortfall. The problem with that thinking was the microeconomics that failed to factor in the declining health of 77 million aging baby boomers that will break the bankrupt debt ceiling that already exists.

Another symptom of the demise of health care as we know it is the demise of the long term care insurance market (see Exhibit A). It is being replaced by managed care, risk pools and capitation payment for the continuum of care called Accountable Care Organizations (ACOs are an academic idea that paying less will enforce more efficiency upon the providers who are grossly ineffective in managing their businesses) . When has enforcement ever resulted in a positive influence in any problem solving endeavor. Read my small nursing home business' P/L statement NEVER.

About $1 trillion will be spent over the next decade on research grants to enhance academic and bureaucratic intellectuals' income—takes resources away from improved outcomes. The ACOs will be funded by the federal government through capitation formulas that take population groups by age and mathematically determine how much will be spent per capita without regard for quality outcomes with incomes based on cutting the cost per capita to a minimum without regard for the impact aging America will have on the high-risk baby boomers.

This takes resources away from true savings programs—the first half of the bill involves a national health-care strategy that we need, and the last half wastes enough on enforcement and a wish list to fund the first half.

Who is going to monitor this monster of regulatory and legalese? It will take sixteen thousand IRS agents, fifty thousand bureaucrats, and one hundred thousand attorneys to figure out how to police and how to game the system while allowing the politicians to control our unhealthy lives.

QUALITY—NOT

Only God knows how the middle class will pay for it: we, the small business owners and taxpayers who already pay *forty-four* different taxes and get no better health-care services.

Do we have a commonsense leader in the country who will stop this lawmaking nightmare and start the elimination of imposing and resource-wasting laws?

WHAT IT DOES NOT TELL THE TAXPAYER

1. Impact of rationing out the dollars on the seven thousand Americans per day reaching sixty-five years of age.
2. How seventy-seven million Americans are going to get their benefits when the trust funds will be insolvent by 2021.
3. Puts regulatory enforcement and restricted innovation to government grants in the hands of the bureaucracy. The Department of Health and Human Services has over twenty-five websites that dictate how the money will be rationed out. Many that are based on the premise of punitive regulatory controls cuts the costs through enforcement, not collaborative and creative enterprise. "You cannot trust the private sector to police its own businesses."
4. Health-care payment currently reimburses for illness, not wellness; medications, hospitalizations, tests, rehospitalizations, ER visits, DRGs, RUGs, RVUs, and OPPS all pay for illness, not wellness.
5. Physicians, hospitals, nurses, therapists, etc., have no standardized processes and think inductively when intervening and establishing care plans.
6. Use of information technology for efficiency requires standardization of terminology and processes to be effective.

7. Best practices will not emerge until we pay for outcomes, not incomes.
8. Why is there only distrust of the private sector to produce better results without infringement on entrepreneurial initiative?
9. It will take creative economic incentives to attain moral incentives, not sixteen thousand IRS auditors and fifteen thousand RAC auditors.

YOU'RE NOT GOING TO LIKE THIS E-MAIL!

At age 76, when you most need it, you are not eligible for cancer treatment.

What Nancy Pelosi didn't want us to know until after the health-care bill was passed was ... she said, Here it is! "Pass it and then read it!"

Obama Care Highlighted by Page Number

THE CARE BILL HB 3200

Judge Kithil is the second official who has outlined these parts of the care bill.

Judge Kithil of Marble Falls, Texas, highlighted the most *egregious* **pages of HB3200.**

Please read this, *especially the reference to pages 58 and 59.*

JUDGE KITHIL wrote:

** Page 50, section 152: The bill will provide insurance to all non-U.S. residents, even if they are here illegally.

** Pages 58 and 59: The government will have real-time access to an individual's bank account and will have the authority to make electronic fund transfers from those accounts.

** Page 65, section 164: The plan will be subsidized (by the government) for all union members, union retirees and for community organizations (such as the Association of Community Organizations for Reform Now—ACORN).

** Page 203, lines 14–15: The tax imposed under this section will not be treated as a tax. [How could anybody in their right mind come up with that?]

** Pages 241 and 253: Doctors will all be paid the same regardless of specialty, and the government will set all doctors' fees.

** Page 272, section 1145: Cancer hospital will ration care according to the patient's age.

** Pages 317 and 321: The government will impose a prohibition on hospital expansion; however, communities may petition for an exception.

** Page 425, lines 4–12: The government mandates advance-care planning consultations. Those on Social Security will be required to attend an "end-of-life planning" seminar every five years. [Death counseling.]

** Page 429, lines 13–25: The government will specify which doctors can write an end-of-life order.

HAD ENOUGH? Judge Kithil then goes on to identify:

> Finally, it is specifically stated that this bill will not apply to members of Congress. Members of Congress are already exempt from the Social Security system, and have a well-funded private plan that covers their retirement needs. If they were on our Social Security plan, I believe they would find a very quick "fix" to make the plan financially sound for their future.

—Honorable David Kithil of Marble Falls, Texas

All of the above should give you the ammo you need to support your opposition to Obamacare.

Please send this information on to all of your e-mail contacts.

A simple bipartisan legislative fix for Obama care would be the following utilizing the current Medicare and Medicaid funds:

1. Federalize Medicaid and take the State waivers out of the politics.
2. Expand Medicare benefits to the different risk pools based on age, health history and weight
3. Use health profiles to set up private and public collaboration for implementation
4. Fund different risk pools: young and healthy, old and healthy, young unhealthy, old unhealthy and rest

5. Different funds: medical, psychiatric, disability, obesity, chronic, unemployed
6. Fund medical from general tax, psychiatric from tax on drugs, disability from tax on business, chronic from tax on seniors, unemployed a Medicaid tax for indigent
7. Integration of Care to be set up by the private sector with the following objectives:

- The continuum of care must be built on processes and models of care and prevention
- The models must be computer generated based on an assessment (diagnosis) of the patient's history and current condition
- The standardized models will be customized to the patient's plan of care
- Cost accounting principles will be utilized for estimating the cost of the episode of care and the expected outcome(s)
- The health care team of physician, nurse, therapist, pharmacist, medical supply custodian and finance team will finalize the care and cost plan
- The length of stay will be estimated and a margin analysis made based on proposed pricing for financial plan
- Execution of the plan by the health care team with benchmarking the cost and the margin during the stay
- Episodic data by ICD-10 code will be captured for trending and metric analysis to validate cost and pricing standards

CHAPTER THREE
HOW GOVERNMENT AND POLITICIANS MONOPSONIZE AND BRUTALIZE SMALL BUSINESSES

Jerry Rhoads' Position Paper on Regulators Retaliation against the Paradigm Shift to Deductive Health Care Economics

Following is my personal experience of calculated retaliation for implementing outcome-based payment and reinforcement surveys in Little Rock, Arkansas, Muscatine, and Washington, Iowa.)

ENFORCEMENT MENTALITY OF GOVERNMENT

ENERGY
NULLIFIED
FOR
OWNERS
RISKING
CAPITAL
EQUITY
MONEY
EGO
NEGATING
TALENT

Enforcement by the bullying government destroys initiative, risk taking, persistence, progress, and freedom of thought for the sake of power and dominance of the enterprising Americans who must start small to be building the bigger infrastructure that creates the environment to make the whole great. The American dream killed by American government is catch 25. Sure you can try, but your effort will die with enforcement.

IS AMERICA BECOMING THE NEXT VERSION OF THE HUNGER GAMES?

According to Suzanne Collins's trilogy *Hunger Games*, after the demise of the games and the revolution against the totalitarian Capitol government for the sake of humanity, there was to be peace on Earth.

The questions are just beginning. The arenas have been completely destroyed, the memorials built, there are no more Hunger Games. But they teach about them at school, and the girl knows we played a role in them. The boy will know in a few years. How can I tell them about a world without frightening them to death? My children, who take the words of the song for granted:

> Deep in the meadow, under the willow,
> A bed of grass, a soft green pillow
> Lay down your head, and close your sleepy eyes
> And when again they open, the sun will rise.
>
> Here it's safe, here it's warm
> Here the daisies guard you from every harm
> Here your dreams are sweet and tomorrow brings them true
> Here is the place where I love you.

Thanks to Suzanne Collins's version of how ordinary victims of oppression can deny the Capitol's totalitarian use of fear, indulgence, and deprivation for inhumane control. By taking what we learn from the Hunger Games, we now have the opportunity to avoid that same struggle by peacefully replacing our government's bureaucratic and regulatory approach to controlling life with common-folk sense for an enterprising, rewarding life. But this requires that the enterprise be a third alternative to our current two-party oppressive (regulatory) games. "Give us enterprise or give us debt, that is our challenge" (*Big Government Rides Again: A True Story of Government Corrupt Intrusion into Enterprise* by Jerry Rhoads).

Timeline for Acquiring Parkview Nursing and Rehabilitation Center, Little Rock, Arkansas: Our First Mistake

Parkview was a client of Jerry Rhoads's consulting business for a period of 2½ years. During that time, there was concern about the facilities management's capabilities, and there was negotiations going on with Edward Holman, operator, and his director of operations regarding our help to deal with regulatory issues and reimbursement implications of being a "special focus" facility. Those negotiations did not lead to any arrangement until a telephone call to Jerry Rhoads in August 2009 from Ed Holman, who indicated he was going to lose the facility license unless it was sold. He suggested that I call Rick Griffin and negotiate a takeover of the lease or purchase the facility.

I called Mr. Griffin and eventually talked to his broker regarding All-American Care Centers Inc., about the purchasing of the facility. I did indicate an interest, and he had Rick Griffin call me direct. Over a period of two to three weeks, we agreed to purchase the facility and work with Mr. Holman to do a transition from him turning over operation to Jerry and his team (Gene Vestal, Kip Rhoads, Jane Vestal, and Shari) to work with the regulators on what they wanted to see happen. CMS had imposed what is termed a *DQIP* and an SIA, agreements that were regulatory remedies to enable All-American Care to assume the provider numbers and continue to receive Medicare and Medicaid funding.

This required that Ed Holman sign the agreements and hand over to All-American Care (AAC) those responsibilities. Effective October 1, 2009, AAC assumed control under a management agreement with a duration related to AAC getting the provider numbers converted, which was effective with them getting a state license that was effective November 1, 2009. On November 24, there was a revisit on the F level violation that was cleared so AAC could be paid. Those payments had to go to the prior operator since the tie process had not been completed, and they were to send us the money for October and thereafter until the tie-in was complete (that did not happen until February 2, 2010). In the meantime, AAC employed Darlene Spinks, former administrator, as the "champion" and Linda Mathis as "nurse consultant," who were assigned the responsibility for complying with the DQIP and SAI systems and procedure for quality improvement.

According to Darlene and Linda, we were in compliance and had met all four of the milestones stipulated in the process and that we were ready for the federal survey. On January 25, the state surveyors started the process and ended on the thirty-first. The state surveyors completed the federal survey and issued ninety-six pages in the 2567 that included an IJ for a van incident (K level of severity went to IDR March 30, and we were told that we did not document the inspection of the seatbelt every day. So the violation, even though we had corrected the problem without incident, did not matter, and we should pay a fine of $10,000 reduced to $6,500 if we don't ask for an ALJ review. We feel this was onerous and did not follow due process of law) and an F level of severity on infection control because of the lack of documentation of follow up on lab tests. This put us in a decertification fast track effective March 5 and to end in closure April 4 unless we decided to self-terminate our Medicare and Medicaid contract and reapply, which we did based on counsel's and CMS's advice.

We had understood that the state would be out shortly after April 4 to do the Medicaid reapplication survey and put us in the reasonable assurance period for the Medicare reapplication. We still do not have any of this happening, and we will run out of money and have to file for bankruptcy unless we get cooperation and help from the state.

Since March 10, we have had seven complaint surveys, cleared six, and the one we did not substantiate was a self-reported elopement, without incident, by the younger sister of our HR director, who walked out with some visitors looking for her sister. We have since found a placement for the sister, who has a locked unit (we feel this is being forced on both sisters).

Since March 4, when the State sent a letter to the families, we have had a decline in census of ten per day from ninety-three to eighty-three and have incurred losses of $100,000 for February and $104,000 for March and over $110,000 for the month of April.

Cash flow—wise, we have borrowed $500,000 from the seller of the business, borrowed $600,000 on a line of credit due to the increase in accounts receivable and are requesting another $600,000 to get us through the reapplication shortfall. Hopefully, this will be enough.

We have asked for AIPP assistance in making sure we pass the Medicaid and Medicare surveys and are following their coaching along with implementing the caregiver-management systems for assigning the work to the staff and documenting outcomes for improving the quality of care.

Postscript

One year later after reapplying for Medicare and Medicaid certification that was earned with only a desk review, we were forced to turn the facility back to the builder; since then, we have been fighting off lawsuits for the costs of turning the facility around to being no. 3 in the market from no. 13 as respectable in a market of punitive regulators and litigious clientele. To date, we have five wrongful death suits pending on patients we don't even acknowledge as being our direct responsibility; this is after the liability insurance lapsed, so as my attorney points out, no good deed ever goes unpunished.

Local Nursing Care Center Fights Back
State of Iowa Regulators Retaliate Against All-American Care of Washington: Our Second Mistake

Facts: An entrepreneur, Jerry Rhoads, is from Iowa originally. He, his wife, and son have returned to Iowa on a mission. It is to change the paradigm for caring for aging Americans from the traditional nursing home to a restorative care center.

They purchased Muscatine Care Center in September 2009, one month before they took over their struggling client in Little Rock, Arkansas, and also converted it to the restorative model of care. The restorative model, invented by the Rhoads family, versus institutional care is like night and day. We all know what the institutions have not been able to do. The restorative model, on the other hand, restores the whole person to their highest level of physical, mental, social, and spiritual functioning.

The Rhoadses have proven in three short years at their Muscatine facility that this model works where the institutional model has not. Using this approach, the Rhoads family has taken an old institutional business, invested $500,000 in renovation to restore dignity, converted antiquated systems to modern computer and security systems to bring quality of care and life to Iowans.

This approach has resulted in many more of the elderly being restored and returned home (57 percent to be exact). Fewer being sent to the hospital ER or beds (less than 17 percent to be exact) and reduced dependency on prescription drugs (33 percent fewer pills). Dramatic results at All-American Care of Muscatine.

The Rhoads family then purchased another failing nursing home in Washington, Iowa, for the purpose of doing the same extreme makeover there. The community is thrilled to have the facility back in the business community. To date, $400,000 has been invested in the renovations on top of the purchase price, and four months later, the facility is becoming respectable.

Now comes the bad news. As in the Muscatine conversion, the inherited policies, procedures, systems, methods have to be upgraded or changed. The staff that is now in a team environment with specific uniforms (nurses in white, not scrubs) have accountability systems directing them. Many don't want change and leave or are terminated. In Muscatine, over 150 employees were replaced or hired for new positions until the right professionals were in place. In the process, the business doubled its revenues and created fifty new jobs.

The same process is being implemented in Washington, but then a disgruntled employee called the State of Iowa Department of Inspections and Appeals hotline with a five-part complaint.

1. Building too cold
2. Staff sleeping at night

3. Incontinent patients not changed timely
4. Baths not given timely
5. Inadequate supervision

Under the enforcement rules followed by the State of Iowa, the provider is guilty until proven innocent. Following is the insanity that small business faces with big government:

1. Anyone anytime can call the state hotline with any trumped-up violation, particularly from a former or current disgruntled employee.
2. State must, by regulations, investigate on-site every complaint.
3. The complainant does not have to inform the facility before calling the state, giving the facility a chance to correct this allegation.
4. State sends a complaint surveyor into the facility unannounced and holds them hostage for days at a time.
5. By regulation, they do not have to inform the facility of who complained, why they complained, and the facility's right to defend themselves.
6. The surveyor is to focus on the complaint stated in the phone call, unless they detect noncompliance elsewhere, and they always do.
7. Violation detection is the objective of the surveyor. Dig and you will certainly find dirt, and they generally do.
8. A report of deficiencies is then issued from the state DIA office after the surveyor gives a noncommittal cursory report to the facility regarding findings before exiting the facility.
9. The higher-ups in Des Moines assign scope and severity codes to each violation with no cross-examination or testimony from the facility and establish punitive allegations, fines, while holding Medicare/Medicaid reimbursement for new admissions forcing the facility into an appeal. The presumed violations are then posted on the DIA website as final, for all to see, two days after the notice is sent to the provider.
10. The facility is given ten days from the date the surprises hit the provider's fax machine or e-mail to garner a defense, if any. Typically, the facility knuckles under and allows this to

go on their eternal record, which can be used against them in later surveys.

Now does that sound like due process of law and compliant with the Administrative Procedure Act? No. That is why I am dredging up this problem, that would be resolved if we could collaborate with the surveyors as we did in Illinois in the 1980s. When the State descends on us that way, it isn't right and is not improving care one inch and has not in the thirty years I have been exposed to it. It is insanity using as punishment working overtime.

Yes, nursing homes, for the most part, have been despicable, smelly, depressing institutions. Most are owned and operated by owners and investors who never go there. (The owners of Muscatine had never been there in thirty years.) Real estate has been the focus of the builders, operators, and well-meaning entrepreneurs. But the real business is the restoration of the elderly and disabled to their highest level of functioning so they can return home. That is the stated objective of the Medicare Law that is violated daily by the federal government's interpretation of what they will not pay for. Typically, the elderly and disabled do not get their entitled one hundred days per spell of illness in skilled-nursing facilities because of big government's denial of payment to the providers. Fear is their tactic, punishment is their method.

The average coverage period for a post hospital Medicare patient is twenty-five to thirty days if therapy is involved, with no extended coverage for skilled nursing restoring function, emotional stability, socialization, and performing home inspections.

Now to the point of this position paper on how big government kills small business. On January 25 (three months after All-American Care took over ownership of Washington Care Center), a complaint surveyor came unannounced with the five-part complaint. And over the next three weeks, off and on (January 26, 30, 31, and February 6 and 7, 2012), he dug in to find everything he could through his five-part porthole. The reason for the investigation is not the issue, even though it wasted everyone's time on unsubstantiated complaints.

In this case, three of the five parts were not substantiated but are on the record books. The other two resulted in F-tag 309 and 323 G and an E severity code 320 being assessed. The G level violations automatically generate fines and withholding of reimbursement until the revisit clears the tags. In this case, the state officials went back to a previous owner's survey results seven months prior and decided to treble the fines, so now the $5,000 becomes $15,000 plus $3,000 for lesser violations, plus $300 per day if the plan of care is not timely. All this gets published, and for all they care, we could be forced out of business before we can finish our conversion.

This does not follow the Administrative Procedure Act or the rule of law. And according to administrative rule of law, the providers are allowed due process for contesting allegations and fines. However, all we are allowed is an informal dispute review (IDR), with very strict limitations as to what we can present.

And now for the worst of it: All-American Care was using security cameras in its facilities as a quality-assurance tool to be able to view staff, patients, visitors, and surveyors' activities for the safely of all. Sounds like the right intention. Well, in this case, it hung us with our own rope because the surveyor got wind of it and viewed twenty-four hours' worth of data over an eight-hour period to look at what was going on while he was not there. It then became his tool for incriminating and misinterpreting an incident he wasn't even there to investigate: falls in the secured unit.

The first incident happened in our locked secure unit for demented and Alzheimer's patients. A behavior-problem patient, who had been banging her head on the wall of her room and ripping the curtains down, was viewed on the video stumbling down the hall toward the nursing station, holding up her arms, apparently talking to the ceiling tile.

She stopped and proceeded to then walk backward until she stumbled and fell backward, hit the base of her head, rubbed it with her hand, rolled over against the wall, and remained there. The patient's documented history is of misbehaving and having a habit of lying on the floor in her room or in her closet and had done this at least three times during the previous two days. In this unit, that is acceptable behavior and is not to be construed automatically as a fall.

So the surveyor viewed the video and requested that they see the whole twenty-four-hour period. Kip Rhoads, the director of operations, agreed to let him view the recorded data, assuming that it would absolve the facility of any wrongdoing. Instead, he calculated that it had been forty-eight minutes before anyone responded to what he was now labeling a fall.

Two CNAs and a nurse were observed coming down the hall and glancing over at the patient, thinking she was all right, then deciding to check her. She had the coping mechanism of lying on the floor in the hall and in her room. They rolled her over and lifted her to her feet. There was no blood, no injury noted, and the staff assumed she was all right.

The patient was only 40 feet down the hall from the nursing station, and the testimony from the two staff that were there was they just thought she was doing what she usually did, lying on the floor. Later, a different CNA found a small bump and blood in her hair from a laceration to the right side of her head. She was taken to the hospital emergency room, and the laceration closed and stapled. Later, she returned from ER that day and was then discharged to the hospital psych ward and never returned.

From that point in the video examination, the surveyor began investigating other falls in the rest of facility and cited additional deficiencies that resulted in a cumulative of two G level violations.

The violation became

1. any patient on the floor constitutes a fall,
2. facility staff neglected to respond to the patient's injury (even though they did not know of her injury),
3. with a known fall, a nurse must assess the patient's condition for injury, call the family and doctor, then perform prescribed interventions. This was not done in this circumstance and

constitutes, according to the surveyor, a life-threatening event that requires a self-report to the State and documentation in the patient's record, with an incident report of the injury and outcome.

We met our responsibility for not responding timely to the patient lying on the floor. It is her right to lay on the floor; however, the staff did respond after deciding that she should be checked, and the director of nursing testified to the surveyor that they did not know this was a fall but acceptable behavior, and the only way the surveyor was able to determine the response time was by clocking the video and staying another three days viewing more video and assessing more allegations and fines. He dug into bathing schedules and documentation and asserted that a patient had not been bathed for nine days but did not accept testimony that this patient habitually refused baths and was given sponge or bed baths in the interim. It was not the facility's procedure to record bed baths on the bath sheet. The very statement that we did not bathe a patient for nine days is not factual, nor can the surveyor prove differently.

Summary

1. New providers are expected to meet a higher standard of care than the previous provider.
2. By rule, the video, being a quality-assurance tool, is to be off-limits to the surveyors. We were led to believe that he wanted to absolve us of any wrongdoing, whereas he used it to incriminate and entrap us for the sake of justifying his three weeks at our facility.
3. A double G level of violations with treble damages is the worst scenario for a quality-assurance tool that we allowed the surveyor to use, in good faith, leaving us to deal with the next bureaucratic step up to an IDR, which warns us that we are not to contest the methods of the survey, the fines, or the allegations unless we have been charged with substandard care.

4. We will appeal and have little legal standing to the enforcement, punitive nature of the regulators charged. We had visions of helping small communities in Iowa to have quality long-term restorative care and do away with the institutional model, but it looks like big government wins again.

5. The most onerous rule is how the regulators have embolden everyone entering the nursing homes business to phone in a complaint ... real or not. Former employees, disgruntled current employees, unhappy families, noncompliant patients, etc. to call in a complaint. We have to post the phone number giving everyone else more authority to run this very difficult business without proof or pursuit of resolution before reporting the complaint. This puts the provider of care on the defensive at all times justified or not and kills initiative and problem solving. Then the bad part is the surveyors show up unannounced and can tear into all records without telling the provider why and dredge up any dirt they want to justify a fine. The word entrapment has been wiped out by their immunity to due process of law.

    The extension of this violation of the operators' constitutional rights they require that management, including the employees, to phone in a reportable incident, true or not within 24 hours of the matter ... if not timely there are harsher remedies available to the enforcers.

    We are not winning the battle of allowing entrepreneur Americans to create jobs and better services and products. It is now a legacy of imposed governmental guidelines that do not even follow the rule of law.

To date, our appeals have been lost or deferred until we give in, but we are contemplating legal action against the State of Iowa and the Department of Health and Human Services for total disregard of the administrative procedures relating to patient care and due process of law. As I write this on November 12, the surveyors have descended on my Muscatine facility for their enforcement tactics. The question is, are we ever going to get it right?

Paradox, paradigm, propaganda, and politics give rise to catch 24 in the nursing-home business where the owners cannot run their own businesses unless they have at least a bachelor's degree and passed the licensed administrator's exam along with one year's experience under an experienced administrator. However, they are legally responsible for everything. If the licensed administrator screws up, the owner gets the blame and loses his business, and the administrator loses his license. This is the reason that most nursing homes are owned by conglomerates that use hired guns and protects their responsibility with insurance, and the influence of an owner being on-site is lost forever.

For example, in Iowa, where Governor Branstad fanaticizes about being the healthiest state in the country, stating he wants a collaborative effort with the providers and move away from a "gotcha" system, in fact, creates catch 25 when he makes no changes in a gotcha system and tells the providers to just comply and all will be good. His hired gun, Rod Roberts, the director of DIA, states we have rules and all the providers need to do is comply with our interpretation of punitive rules and civil money penalties.

No matter, because their interpretation is subjective, arbitrary, and capricious based on who you are and how much you pay into their PAC for the next election.

Such is the insanity of ruling by power, not reason, claiming to do good and fix the problems while creating fear and confusion on rules that cannot be met if you are the target of retaliation and contempt using the media and Internet to seek and destroy under the guise of being the healthiest state in the country.

CHAPTER FOUR

ENTERPRISE'S FIRST MOVE: LINK INCOME TO OUTCOME

Why would it result in apparent retaliation? It is the dirtier part of politics.

I invited the governor of Iowa, Terry Branstad, to visit our restorative model of care. He toured, and I gave him white papers on pay for performance and reinforcement surveys and my book *Remedy Eldercide, Restore Elderpride*. I followed up with David Heaton in the legislature and Rod Roberts, director of Inspections and Appeals. This was in July and August 2011, and we purchased Washington Care Center October 11, 2011, and we were buried by the surveyor in January 2012 and throughout 2012 and 2013 with visits, revisits, fines, and hold on admissions five months out of twelve that virtually put us out of business. I cannot get an attorney to take on the state for violating due process of law and the individual's rights of the owners, patients, and families due to immunity and jurisdiction for such treatment.

Then came the help of two legislators, Mark Lofgren and Lance Horbach, who were touting our software programs and operating methods as being a way for the State to improve the care in nursing homes and collaborate rather than punish facilities for alleged violations.

Following are the white papers presented to the governor and director of DIA.

LINK INCOME TO OUTCOME
(Reimburse for Results) White Paper
by Jerry L. Rhoads, CPA, FACHCA

The authors of *Freakonomics* assert that "we all want to believe in the pursuit of moral incentives, but economic incentives are the way things are". America's enterprising economy is built on this reality. Then why is Health Care built on fear, punitive damages, civil penalties, allegations of fraud and abuse to attain what the academics have defined as our moral incentives.

For example the Iowa case mix system for paying for Medicaid nursing care services uses a Minimum Data Set that triggers 19 functional deficits and focuses on activities of daily living not functionality nor restoring the patients' emotional well being nor socialization nor incentives for discharge. This treatment driven reimbursement system does not establish a foundation for economic incentives using outcomes.

At our Muscatine facility the case mix system is destroying our incentive to restore patients back to their highest level of functioning prior to our acquiring the facility the case mix score averaged 1.02 and the rate was a miserable $102 per day and after the recent adjustments that rate rose to $129 with $5 going back to the State for gaming the CMS formula for revenue sharing. Now we just got our case mix score and it is .88 and our rate is going down by $5. The reason for the reduction is we discharged over 50% of our admissions back into the community by reducing their dependence on staff and were scored at higher levels of functioning and guess what? Our rate goes down. This is clearly a bad way to pay.

In addition there are no economic incentives for getting the patients their entitled Medicare benefits before putting them on spend down and then Medicaid. Nationally, CMS has intimidated providers to the point that the average coverage period for Skilled patients is less than 35 days of the 100 they have paid for. As a result the providers take them off because CMS has narrowly interpreted the rules for enforcing the Medicare insurance policy. The policy clearly defines what CMS is to pay for but they categorically ignore the rules. In 1986 HEW was sued and lost in Federal court, *Fox v. Bowen*, for doing the same thing and since then HCFA and CMS buried that case and continue to threaten providers to take the patients off coverage based on their narrow and illegal interpretation of the insurance policy. That policy has not changed because we all are paying for the coverage that most do not get.

The economic impact of this enforcement tactic is to force the skilled nursing facilities to stop therapies after 30 days and leave the patients still unable to function at their highest level for which they have paid for. What then happens costs the health care system $400 billion with more and more of the elderly being warehoused in the nursing homes that CMS asserts as being the bad guys. On the other hand the nursing facilities are not providing restorative services and the patients are relegated to institutions for the rest of their lives.

WHAT IS THE PROBLEM WITH CURRENT REIMBURSEMENT?

As a consultant to the Federal Government and the State of Illinois I wrote the white paper for HEW in 1977 for prospective payment based on acuity and the delivery of restorative services payable first by Medicare then private resources and last resort Medicaid. That proposed method of payment was utilized for establishing the MDS and the use of minutes of care for payment but it was narrowed down to the point that it pays for keeping patients impaired and dysfunctional; no economic incentives exist for discharge or improved functioning at home or in a nursing home.

The MDS form is inadequate to be the basis for determining acuity and the RUGs II, III and IV are only averaging formulas that do not relate to services actually rendered let alone outcomes. Without a valid formula for payment the assisted living industry has entered the scene and is systematically spending down private resources promising a better outcome until the resident's functioning declines and in need of more professional nursing. Ironically given enough time these businesses will turn into nursing homes and have the same outcomes that now exist. We also have the ideas of the Little Green Houses and the Medical Homes to take the nursing homes out of the continuum and try to shift the financial responsibility to the families. We are not solving the problem; we pay for treatment, not outcomes. In fact CMS and its academic approach to all initiatives, because they do not trust the private sector, is proposing more enforcement and less payment for true outcomes.

HOW SHOULD WE PAY?

Payment for outcome rather than income is completely defined in my book *Remedy Eldercide, Restore Elderpride* (you don't know what you don't know). In summary it proposes the following structure and formulas:

- Pay a base rate for room and board based on a cost report updated to current costs
- Pay for add-on programs (contracted rates based on competitive pricing offered by providers to the payment agencies)
    - Physical rehabilitation (gross motor and strengthening skills)
    - Occupational rehabilitation (fine motor and cognitive skills)
    - Social rehabilitation (communication and living skills)
    - Psychological rehabilitation (emotional and decision making skills)
    - Nutritional rehabilitation (weight control and healthy eating skills)
    - Discharge planning (every admit has a plan for discharge to lower levels)
- Pay an annual economic incentive using the QUIP formula proposed in the "Pursuit of Outcomes" paper

HOW MUCH WILL THIS COST THE CURRENT BUDGET?

The major cost for Health Care (Medicare and Medicaid) is re-hospitalization and inappropriate medication usage in nursing homes. Using the payment for Outcome rather than Income will reduce the need to re-hospitalize at a cost $166 billion, if we restore our elderly and the reduction of prescription drug abuse imposed on the unwitting elderly by phone orders from physicians that heap more and more pills on symptoms. Eight billion pills are passed in our nursing homes each year at a cost of $169 billion wasting away our elderly and our ability to get 50% of those souls back into the community under the responsibility of the families rather than State and Federal Government.

HOW MUCH WILL THIS SAVE ABOVE AND BEYOND CURRENT COSTS?

Seventy-seven million baby boomers are coming at health care providers as a demanding tsunami with no plan or preparation with the promise that we will cover everyone for everything. It will take another 20,000 nursing homes over the next 2 decades to handle this unhealthy group unless we

- Restore those that decline before they have to go to the ER or the hospital
- Offer pre-acute care services in our 16,000 nursing homes and pay economic incentives for discharge back to the community based services
- Offer post-acute care services in our 16,000 nursing homes and pay economic incentives for discharge back to the community based services
- Do not bundle reimbursement but let enterprising Americans price and provide the services that innovate new methods not more regulations that do not work (regulators stifle the American spirit for solving problems; let us have economic incentives to accomplish the moral incentives we all want)!
- Reduce medication usage by 33% and use rehab and restorative services for health preservation at the community level as well as congregate solutions.
- Chronic disease costs the current health care system 80% of the resources in the last 2 years of our lives; it is all reactionary and more than likely caused by over use of drugs, poor eating

habits and the lack of incentives for restoring the elderly to their highest level of functioning as they decline not after.
- The use of computer technology can reduce the costs and mistakes currently being imposed on our elderly; by standardizing processes and vernacular so the providers are on the same page not just in a treatment mode but in a continuum of care preventing further decline and preserving health at the earliest age.
- Require, through withholding from paychecks, that each working American have a long term care insurance policy with a health savings account managed by mutual health insurance companies that reinvest the capital in the American economy.

These are enterprise solutions not political theories that have failed us since Blue Cross promised that those covered do not have to worry because the private sector would cover the costs. Now we are buried by that philosophy and it is sinking the American economy.

WHAT ARE THE ALTERNATIVES TO COMPREHENSIVE CHANGE?

The Democrats' Health Care Reform act that just passed Congress that will be repealed if the Republicans have their way is heaping more weight on the American businesses with no reduction in inappropriate costs and promises that we cannot keep that is incremental change. Comprehensive change can happen if the 50 Governors collectively support a plan that will work the payment for outcomes so we all can pursue incomes legitimately by providing restorative services not reactive treatment.

HOW CAN WE ACCOMPLISH THIS COMPREHENSIVE CHANGE?

If New York City was going to be flooded by Niagara Falls and 6 million people would die could we redirect the deluge? Would we incrementally strive to redirect it or would we prevent the flooding? I propose yes turn off the faucet and redirect the flow of the destruction. Health Care is not different; turn off the reimbursement flow and pay for performance. We do not have the time to do the piece meal approach and hope that it works. We have to get enterprise involved and redirect how the resources are spent using the above formulas. The Governors must be the catalyst since Congressional and Legislative lawmakers are playing to the special interests not the Good of America.

CHAPTER FIVE

HOW ENTERPRISE HEALTH CARE WINS THE MONOPSONY GAME

Pursuit of Outcomes (a Six-Star Survey) White Paper
Jerry L. Rhoads, CPA, FACHCA

Deepak Chopra, says "if you go there in your mind you will go there in your body"

- Why do health care providers get paid on input units of production rather than output units
- We must go to re-enforcement surveys so our body of work will go for outcomes.
- Currently enforcement looks for mistakes and threatens retaliation if the plan of correction is not completed in 10 days and implemented the next 30 days for a revisit and loss of certification and reimbursement lingers there at all times.
- Threats only get results for a short time. And then are those the right results?
- Re-enforcement and coaching had been found by the great behavioral psychologists to work much better in the long run.

Health Care is Inductive in its Quality Standards/Measures and the Payment Processes (paid on input units) not Deductive (paid on outcome units measuring results):

- Hospitals are paid on DRGs, diagnosis related groups (payment and quality incentives are paid on diagnoses not outcome results)
- Physicians are paid on RVUs, relative value units (payment and quality measures are paid on treatment encounters not on outcome results)

- Nursing homes are paid on RUGs, resource-utilization groups (payment and quality measures are paid on treatments not on outcome results); if you get them better your rate goes down
- Home Care Providers are paid on OASIS, outcome and assessment information set (payment and quality measures are paid on assessment not on outcome results)
- Outpatient Services are paid on OPPS, outpatient perspective payment system (payment and quality measures are paid on treatment not on outcome results)

Why would the biggest business in the world be paid differently than all other businesses who must provide a quality outcome to have income, while health care providers get paid whether they provide a quality product or service referred to an outcome or a positive result? Because the providers are happy not to be held responsible for results and the Government wants to control the flow or resources so it does not have to prove a benefit just a contribution to the cost that they discount because the cost is too high. Providers do not want to be administratively accountable to outcome standards because they would have to define their products and services in relation to their costs per outcome unit which they have never been required to do. Walla, the reason for escalating costs and deteriorating quality of life results.

Re-enforcement has the following attributes:

1. The goal is to look for the good and correct the bad in a collaborative system.
2. Council to remove the defects using outcome driven care planning and programmatic interventions timed to comprehensive assessment instrument.
3. Focus on the problems and solutions pursuing outcomes.
4. Measure progress against the base line goal for each problem (outcomes).
5. Problem, Intervention, Evaluation of the outcomes put a structure to the exercise
    a. Problems assessment is comprehensive not minimal data
    b. Interventions are for programmatic solutions

c. Evaluation of the results are for resolving patient problems using numerical scales
   i. The physical
   ii. The emotional
   iii. The social
   iv. The spiritual

6. **Outcomes pursued**
   a. Reduce readmissions to hospital ER and critical care
   b. Increase discharges back to community based programs and home placements
   c. Reduce inappropriate medications (antidepressants, antibiotics, psychotropics, and PRNs)
   d. Reduce dependency on wheelchairs with more fitness and wellness focus through therapies and restorative programming
   e. Eliminate or reduce negative outcomes using positive incentives
      i. Falls
      ii. Odors
      iii. Dehydration
      iv. Skin breakdown
      v. Neglect
      vi. Loss of dignity
      vii. Physical or emotional Abuse
   f. Promote positive behaviors with incentives for improving
      i. Staff morale, retention, attendance
      ii. Staff pride
      iii. Career plans for advancement
      iv. Learning from problem resolution
         Developing skills that prevent problems

7. **Six stars of quality attained**
   a. 1st Star—environment
   b. 2nd Star—programming for patient condition and productive living
   c. 3rd Star—Documentation by assessed problems of interventions and outcomes

d. 4th Star—Family involvement
e. 5th Star—Community involvement and discharge planning
f. 6th Star—Improved functionality of patients to their highest level for discharge to lowest level of cost with emphasis on home placement

8. **QUIP (Quality Incentive Payment)** (moral incentives are what we would like to attain but economic incentives are the way to get there)
   a. Annual survey to find facilities doing the pursuit of outcomes correctly
   b. Use re-enforcement and coaching to attain the prescribed outcomes
   c. Pay for performance
      i. Base rate for room and board (value added cost of hospitality component = $100 per patient per day)
      ii. Add-on programs (small group restorative programming)
         1. Physical rehab ($5 per day per patient for documented programs)
         2. Occupational rehab ($5 per day per patient for documented programs)
         3. Social rehab ($2 per day per patient for groups of 6 or less)
         4. Psychological rehab ($2 per day per patient for groups of 6 or less)
         5. Spiritual rehab ($1 per day per patient for groups of 10 or less)
         6. Successful Discharge plans ($1500 for each discharge to community)
            a. Typical Medicaid patient would be in 3 physical and occupational rehab programs daily 6 days per week = $90 per week or $13 per day
            b. Typical Medicaid patient would be in 3 psycho/social programs per 7 days per week = $42 per week or $14 per day

c. Spiritual rehab would be 1 day per week = $1 per day
d. Base rate of $100 plus $13, $14, $1 = a billing of $128 per day for each patient in this routine, plus $1500 for each discharge patient to the community based options
e. Billing would be done monthly for the base rate and programming supported by documentation required by patient to support programs and outcomes based on scales for improved deficits (0 to 4 Schedule G assessed function deficits for staff support and patient functionality):
iii. QUIP bonus based on the 6 stars ($1 per Medicaid patient day paid retroactively at the end of the fiscal year for each star attained) 100 bed facility at 80% occupancy = 25,000 X 70% Medicaid = 17,500 incentive days
1. Star = $17,500 incentive payment
2. Stars = $35,000 incentive payment
3. Stars = $52,500 incentive payment
4. Stars = $68,000 incentive payment
5. Stars = $85,500 incentive payment
6. Stars = $103,000 incentive payment (designated as best facilities in the State of Iowa with publicized and trophies displayed)

9. Overall Outcome:
   a. Improved patient care in a holistic environment
   b. Lowest cost of labor due to improved productivity and retention
   c. Fewer re-hospitalizations and use of inappropriate medications

10. Estimated financial impact on a 100 bed facility
    a. Current occupancy 85%
    b. Current turnover rate of staff 89%
    c. Current re-hospitalization rate 4 per year per patient

d. Cost of underutilized capacity = $1.1 million *
e. Cost of staff turnover = .5 million **
f. Cost of re-hospitalization = 8.5 million ***
*15% under utilization of capacity = 5,495 billable days @ $200 per day
** 100 employees with 89 new hires @$5,000 new hire
*** 85 patients x 2 readmits = 170 x$50,000 hospital charges = $8.5 mil

1. Estimated impact nationally of this scenario $10.1 million x 16,000 skilled nursing facilities = $166 billion wasted due to using enforcement rather than re-enforcement in the State of Iowa for 282 skilled facilities = $300 million in Medicare and Medicaid dollars. Contrast enforcement with re-enforcement:
2. Enforcement: the act of compelling observance of or compliance with a law, rule, or obligation. "the strict enforcement of health care regulations regardless of the implications".
3. Re-enforcement: the process of encouraging or establishing a belief or pattern of behavior, especially by encouragement or reward. "the collaborative compliance with health care regulations, resulting in quality of life of the patients in the care of nursing homes".

You tell me ... which will get the better results. That is all I asked for when I met with Rod Roberts the head of Iowa's Department of Inspections and Appeals after my appeal was denied... of course he ignored my plea and pulled Catch 23 on me. "Jerry you can appeal or just comply".

11. The Re-enforcement program was utilized by the State of Illinois from 1985 to 1991 under Republican administration. Add-ons and QUIP were a great success for the performing facilities and the 6 star facilities were the best but the worst has more political power and had it killed. So goes the current money driven health care system.

Shift the Paradigm to Pay for Performance:

Pay the Providers on meeting maximum standards not minimum standards so they pay fewer efficient staff more for providing quality work, rather than more staff less for whatever they decide to do or not do.

CHAPTER SIX

HOW GOVERNMENT MONOPSONY HEALTH CARE SINS

GIVE ME MINIMUM STANDARDS, AND I WILL GIVE YOU MINIMAL CARE

Current Minimum Regulatory Standards for Skilled-Nursing Facilities That Promotes Mediocrity

- 37.106.601 Minimum Standards for a Skilled-Nursing Care Facility—General
- 37.106.605 Minimum Standards for a Skilled-Nursing Care Facility—Staffing
- 37.106.606 Minimum Standards for a Skilled-Nursing Care Facility—Prescription Drugs
- 37.106.640 Minimum Standards for a Skilled-Nursing Care Facility—Infirmary
- 37.106.645 Minimum Standards for a Skilled-Nursing Care Facility –Developmentally Disabled
- 37.106.650 Minimum Standards for a Skilled-Nursing Care Facility—Kidney Treatment

Presently, control is futilely trying to be attained through threats, penalties, fear tactics and less reimbursement. In my opinion, this approach makes care worse. It does not deal with the problem; it deals with symptoms. Poor care is due to lack of economic incentives to provide a quality of life for those who are forced to accept the alternative lifestyle in nursing facilities—and there is not any educational training to assist nursing-facility providers in improvement; the government and the provider are at opposite ends, a "we against them" scenario, using subjective intimidation, as opposed to a more democratic environment where both the government and providers are working together to achieve quality care.

It is not the patient's desired home, and the staff needs stability, not threats; organization and process development and control, not more people; tools for efficiency, not more hours; models of care designed to address problems and achieve goals, not guessing on what should be done; and more involvement with the medical community, not a cursory visit by a physician every thirty days skilled and ninety days nonskilled with phone orders galore.

A PROPOSAL FOR MAXIMUM STANDARDS That Reward Excellence

The cliché "Minimum standards become maximum quality" certainly applies in many nursing homes. Since there are no incentives to do better than minimum, there are no reasons to exceed what you have to provide to minimally pass a subjective survey process, rather than a survey process based on factual data.

Survey happens once a year, around contract renewal dates, so it is *supposed* to be totally a surprise visit. The surveyors are typically former nursing employees who are allowed to subjectively interpret the minimum standards during their visit.

Nursing-home management is given ten days to develop a plan of correction for those violations noted by the surveyors and the fire marshall. If the plan is accepted, the State has the option for doing a follow-up survey or accept the correction plan through a desk review.

Nursing-home reforms have been promulgated and directed toward additional or revised deficiencies for years. However, very few facilities are held financially accountable for providing quality outcomes, which can be reviewed from statistical and factual data.

What would be the maximum standards?

- 37.106.601 Maximum Standards for a Skilled-Nursing Care Facility—General. A facility that is clean, without odors, and provides adequate space for patients, families, and visitors would receive one of six stars of quality.

- 37.106.605 Maximum Standards for a Skilled-Nursing Care Facility—Staffing. A facility that utilizes care plans for determining the amount of staff based on the care plans would receive one of six stars of quality.
- 37.106.606 Maximum Standards for a Skilled-Nursing Care Facility—Pharmaceuticals. A facility that institutes a drug-reduction program involving attending physicians and pharmacies would receive one of six stars of quality.
- 37.106.640 Maximum Standards for a Skilled-Nursing Care Facility—Hospitalization. A facility that reduces the incidences of rehospitalization by at least 25 percent each year receives one of the six stars of quality.
- 37.106.645 Maximum Standards for a Skilled-Nursing Care Facility—Dementia and Alzheimer's. A facility that institutes psychosocial programming receives one of the six stars of quality.
- 37.106.650 Maximum Standards for a Skilled-Nursing Care Facility—Activities of Daily Living Optimized. A facility that institutes restorative and retraining programs for all patients receives one of six stars of quality.

This six stars of quality, based on maximum standards, would replace the meaningless five-star program promulgated by CMS, based on minimum standards (see Chapter 15 for the proposed change to the ineffective, harmful CMS' 5 star program),

SIX STARS TO SUCCESSFUL QUALITY

The only system that has been developed that works is the Illinois six star system for skilled nursing facilities (I refer to this in my books). It was implemented with my help in the 1980's by the Department of Public Health and was called the QUIP program. It measures results not input units of mistakes and inaccurate metrics for quality of care and life. The six stars was an annual survey in six areas of outcome where the surveyors measured performance on those criteria that could be defined as contributing to the patients' welfare and functionality.

- First star = care planning and staff effectiveness
- Second star = documentation of attaining goals for problems
- Third star = family involvement and satisfaction
- Fourth star = Community and volunteer involvement
- Fifth star = productive activities and psycho/social programming
- Sixth star = discharge planning

The corresponding reimbursement system then paid for the add-on programs of restorative care that generated the six star results. It then paid an economic incentive for each star earned and paid retroactive bonuses based on that collaborative accountability system. Therefore, the six star facilities were truly the best in the state. I took over two no star facilities and turned them around by focusing the staff on attaining the six stars. Those providers who did not attain that status were incentivized to pursue each star and become the best. This system was thrown out by the Illinois Legislature because the big noncompliant owners did not want that accountability and distinction as a one or two star facility. This system works.

For example, a guest column in a New Jersey community paper called the *Sentinel*. "Ten qualities of a great nursing home" was written by Fern Marder, who happens to be the marketing communications manager for Parker Homes, which is based in the Garden State.

For the record, she notes that great facilities offer:

- A sense of community
- A comfortable environment
- A home-like atmosphere
- Person-centered living
- Around-the-clock skilled care
- Outdoor spaces
- Meaningful activities
- Excellent food that's nutritious
- Anytime visitation
- Amenities such as hair salons/barber shops, health and wellness centers and libraries.

The current CMS five star program does not measure success only failure.

- Quality measures – metrics that measure mistakes not results
- Health inspections - Survey results one and a half years old
- Staffing and number of RN's
- Cumulative

I CALL THE SIX STARS - HUMAN TECHNOLOGY

My definition of human technology is "get along better with what you have" and "get rid of things that are not necessary to the outcome then team up and get out of the way of change". The reason is to turn an organizational nightmare into a science (the science of managing human value) which I call Mancology. The equation is $E3 = C + F \times T$ (efficiency/effectiveness/excellence equals creativity plus focus times human technology). This is a systemic change in operational management, not just a policy change in HR.

- Create the environment for change
- Focus staff interventions on priorities
- Use human technology to direct the process and account for quality
- And change the outcome to efficiency and effectiveness of the human asset

In my experience this will raise morale, raise productivity, raise quality and that raises profits…because the hidden wasteful costs go down…unwanted turnover goes away…unapproved absences cease. This is a form of Six Sigma in that it is the result of human technology not the reason for it. The reason is human beings aiding other human beings.

Humanity existence consists of the visual, the nano physical, the meta physical and the neo physical experiences, as does technology. So the impact of the underlying nano physical, meta physical and neo physical are where the extreme human performance advances coexist.

They are interconnected and cohesive. They hold existence together and provide stability.

What does this mean in reality? We now know that we can communicate digital information at electronic nano speeds and that creates a nano physical function and a meta-physical phenomena called efficiency and knowledge…but does it make the result more real more permanent. No it does not until the neo physical is put into the equation…that is the personal side of the equation…what does this efficiency and knowledge mean to me…the neo person.

Example: I met a guy at a hotel in Columbus, Ohio…we were watching the Bulls championship game and commenting on how the great teams work. He asked me why I was there and I said to put on a seminar for nursing homes on team, management…he replied "that is a coincidence so am I"…his story goes like this…the National Chamber of Commerce had hired him to put on seminars around the country on his management method because of his success…he was almost embarrassed when he told me his story…according to him his business in Cedar Rapids, Iowa was going south…he was so fed up with it that he decided to take two weeks off and turned the keys over to the employees…when he came back in two weeks there was a dramatic improvement in getting things done…so much so he decided to take two months off…came back and the business was now making money and stable…so much so he took another six months off and another and another; that was his way of improving efficiency, productivity, effectiveness and profitability…that method is "get along better with what you have" and, "get rid of things that are not necessary (usually middle or ineffective managers) team up and get out of the way of change".

Human technology therefore must consist of the following:

1) Obvious physical changes
2) Metabolic changes in human function
3) Needed psychological changes
4) Created social changes
5) Experienced spiritual changes

6) Shared outcomes or actualizing by making a difference in lives

All this can be accomplished in three days by just leaving it up to the teams that know the business to figure out how to implement higher quality and lower or eliminate waste. The Japanese did it following an American's formula...so why not American health Care using it for real change.

For example a nursing home is remodeled and made more physically enticing so it smells better looks better appears better...but the staff still does not show up for work on schedule and the morale is not good...that psychological change has not taken place because the changes did not include better organizational improvements such as adding tools for gaining efficiency and capability to get the important things done...physical technology will make the social changes happen because the staff now has time to socialize with the patients and gain a personal relationship that helps both the person and the patient be spiritually connected. Metabolically the staff and patient grow and attain better neo physical outcomes if human technology is implemented.

How can this connection happen and allow the human technology to be embraced to support the computer technology, the physical technology of better equipment and better environmental changes for nutritional and fitness. It has to be a neo physical change...that entails a change in priorities from money to outcome from income to using human technology to improve human morale and human performance.

Human technology consists of:

1) Functional management
2) Team organization
3) Blue prints of care – evidence based actions standardized care models
4) Case managers and electronic case management systems
5) Pursuit of outcome (P.I.E.)

6) Measurement of performance
7) Reward excellence (QUIP)

Functional management:

Define the function and you have defined the job. It is not CNA or RN those are titles not functions. The function is defined by the patients' needs:

1) Activities of Daily living
2) Medical instability
3) Mental instability
4) Social instability
5) Psychological instability

Match the function with the need:

1) CNA, RA, SA, Hospitality Aide for the ADL's instability
2) MD, RN's, LPN's, PT, OT, ST, LPTA, COTA, for medical instability
3) CSW, Psychiatrist for mental instability
4) Activity, recreational and religious for social instability
5) RN, LPN, CNA, RA, SA, CSW, Psychiatrist for mental instability

Match the care plan with the patient's need:

- Symptoms (clinical assessment)
- Cause (clinical analysis)
- Diagnosis (medical conclusion of cause)
- Problem definition (ADL, medical, mental, social, psychological)
- Intervention (skilled, personal services, hospitality services)
- Goals (baseline deficit scales, outcome deficit scales, progress deficit scales)
  - 4 = totally dependent
  - 3 = extensive assistance needed
  - 2 = limited assistance needed

- o 1 = supervision needed
- o 0 = totally independent

Team Organization:

Specialize teams based on Instabilities

- Medical
    - o Post hospital rehab – therapists, rehab aides,
    - o Transitional Care – therapists, rehab aides
    - o Chronic Care – restorative aides

- Mental
    - o Reality care – CSW's, social services aides
    - o Dementia care – CSW's, social services aides
    - o Alzheimer's care – CSW's, social services aides

- Social
    - o Emotional management – CSW's, social services aides
    - o Wandering – CSW's, social services aides
    - o Communication – CSW's, social services aides
    - o Recreational – Social Therapists, Activity aides
    - o Wellness and fitness - therapists, rehab aides, restorative aides

- Psychological
    - o Behavior management – CSW's, social services aides
    - o Depression management – CSW's, social services aides
    - o Co-dependencies – CSW's, social services aides
    - o Addictions – CSW's, social services aides

- ADL – CNA's, RA's
    - o Ambulation
    - o Strengthening
    - o Dressing
    - o Clothing
    - o Eye glasses, dentures and hearing aides
    - o Bathing

- o Eating
- o Grooming
- o Transfer
- o Bed mobility
- o Wheel chair safety

Case Management and electronic case management systems:

- Every patient is a case
- Every episode is a case action
- Every problem is a case action
- Case Managers have a case load
- Case Managers have a case management team
- Case Managers have a case management system for implementing the care plan based on the patients assessed problems, needs and expected outcomes
- Case Management software Systems employee time values for the care plan interventions, frequency of the interventions, duration of the interventions so the labor costs can be forecast and controlled. Activity based costing and acuity staffing are calculated from this data base.

Pursuit of Outcome (P.I.E. problem assessment, interventions and evaluation of outcome):

- Base line assessed level of deficit 0 to 4
- Base line assessed level of pain, vital signs, skin turgor, confusion, etc., i.e. a statistical measurement is required to manage the pursuit of improvement or stopping decline or managing the dying process
- Expected level of outcome by problem stated as goals (improvement, palliative, sustenance, or preventive)

Measurement of Performance:

- Measuring progress or decline of the patient's condition should be numerical so the trends over time over different cases with similar diagnosis and/or problems can be analyzed.

- Measuring staff's effectiveness is better served if that person is on a team for a particular function then we can track results for that person for that patient for that day…performance for the staff can be measured in time for efficiency and in the condition of the patient for the team…but for the individual staff position it relates to their particular function…i.e., prevention of bed sores, patient's ability to dress self, ambulate without a device, communicate room # and day of the week.
- Quality of the care or the quality of life for the patient is a longer term goal and outcome…if more can function without a wheelchair and take fewer medications those are measurable and very positive…but getting out of diaper and being continent may take longer and vary from day to day. If the team is structured around function there is a way to measure effectiveness…if the position is CNA and the function is tracking eyeglasses, dentures and hearing aides effectiveness is the number of lost items that are found or replaced the day they are lost…if it goes beyond a day the likely hood of it being found is remote and replacement becomes the measure of effectiveness.
- The ultimate measure I found was how many problem makers can I turn into problem solvers and how many problems do they solve at the lowest level without management's intervention.

Reward Excellence (QUIP or in Governmental parlance pay 4 performance)

1) How many admissions are transitioned back to the community
2) How many post hospital patients are restored to their highest level of ADL functioning
3) How many patients were weaned off tubes, psychotropic drugs, blood thinner, cholesterol medication, anti anxiety drugs, diapers wheelchairs
4) How many of our CNA's become nurses
5) How many of our hospitality aides become CNA's and/or RA's
6) How many of our social services designees become CSW's

7) How many of our dietary workers become Aides
8) Payment for hotel services should be a base rate plus the following add-ons for rehab and restorative programs:
   a. Physical rehab add-on
   b. Occupational rehab add-on
   c. Social rehab add-on
   d. Speech rehab add-on
   e. Restorative nursing add-on
   f. Psycho/social add-on
   g. Quality incentive payment (QUIP)

Summary:

When I took over Fox Valley, a 207 bed skilled nursing facility, we had 175 employees that did not want to work there, 175 patients that did not want to be there and 175 families who did not want to come there...plus Fox Valley had been decertified and I had operational breakdowns every day as a result of that situation.

It took a drowning in the whirlpool, a breakdown in the air conditioning system and a 3 day blizzard to bring salvation to roost... out of desperation we formed teams and discarded the departmental organization, organized like-problem patients in the same area, focused our care on their specialized needs, used the care plan as the assignment and accountability device and cleaned up the mess. The rest is history.

The transition in staff morale, which is the most important ingredient in any change, happened over the three day week-end snow storm and we never looked back...so we did in three days what I am told by the industry can't be done at all. That is what I call human technology... when you can do something in three days that is called impossible.

After the use of human technology we had 200 patients that were glad to be there, 175 employees that liked working there and 200 families that would come there...that is evidence based and performance measured skilled nursing care. $E3 = C + F \times T$

CHAPTER SEVEN

HOW ENTERPRISE HEALTH CARE LOSES

Since I have not been able to engage an attorney to take on their friends at the State of Iowa and/or DIA, due to legal immunity, following are the allegations I plan to take to court pro se (my own counsel) for a new form of justice that holds the bureaucrats accountable for destroying small business and the very passion that makes a difference.

UNITED STATES DISTRICT COURT
—The Lawsuit That Needs to be Heard by the Public and Private Interests in Pursuit of Health Care Reform
DISTRICT OF IOWA

PLAINTIFF: JERRY L. RHOADS, ATTORNEY PRO SE.

v.

Department Director
Rodney A. Roberts
Division Administrator
Dawn Fisk
Medicare/Medicaid Bureau I
Assistant Division Administrator
Kathy Sutton, Bureau Chief
Medicare/Medicaid Bureau II
Mindla White, Bureau Chief
Medicare/Medicaid Bureau III
Kathy Kieler, Bureau Chief
Complaint/Incident Bureau
Joni Klaassen, Bureau Chief
Compliance Officers
Donna Spencer
Hema Lindstrom

Case No.:

COMPLAINT FOR DECLARATORY AND INJUNCTIVE RELIEF

Southeast Iowa
Donna Walters, Program
Coordinator
Complaint/Incident Bureau
Joni Klaassen, Bureau Chief
Geri Paul, Program Coordinator
Abuse Coordinating Unit
Stephanie Jones, Program
Coordinator
Rob Reck, RN Surveyor

**DES MOINES *REGISTER* AND
CLARK KAUFFMAN
COLLECTIVELY AND
INDIVIDUALLY
400 Locust Street, Suite 500
Des Moines, IA, 50309
    Defendants.**

COMPLAINT FOR DECLARATORY AND INJUNCTIVE RELIEF

Now comes plaintiff Jerry L. Rhoads, part owner of two skilled-nursing facilities in the State of Iowa, which, for their complaint against defendants, state as follows:

PRELIMINARY STATEMENT

1. This is an action brought by Jerry L. Rhoads, part owner with his wife and son (also individual plaintiffs pro se) of the All-American Care of Muscatine and Washington, hereunder referred to the provider or the owners to permanently enjoin defendants from making "arbitrary rules" and cease and desist from capriciously applying public health standards in conducting their surveys of nursing facilities not taking into consideration extenuating circumstances in applying the rule of law and due process as it applies to skilled-nursing facilities. This resulting in an intentional disregard for the

Administrative Procedure Act as it relates to retaliatory tactics against the provider, defaming the owners, utilizing the Internet for punishment before the appeal process has been exhausted, using complaint surveys to expand the intended investigation into all areas of the operation with the intent to compile and exaggerate allegations that result in civil money penalties and remedies exerted by CMS to the damage of the owners, the business, and the patients, and above all, using the media to punish providers who are at most times innocent of such extreme treatment. And requiring that the providers self-incriminate using the self-report and complaint tactics for generating civil money penalties, fines, and harmful holds on admitting patients under the criminal aspect of the statute. These tactics are well known by the industry as being arbitrary and capricious without fair representation by counsel or the associations and are applied subjectively across the board and are corrupt in their very nature.

JURISDICTION

2. The court has jurisdiction over this action pursuant to 28 U.S.C. §§1331 and 1343, in that plaintiff is seeking declaratory and injunctive relief under 28 U.S.C. §2201 and 2202.
3. This court may enter a declaratory judgment as provided in 28 U.S.C. §2201 and federal rule of civil procedure 57. Injunctive relief may be granted as provided by federal rule of civil procedure 65.

VENUE

4. Venue is proper in this district pursuant to 28 U.S.C. §1391(b) and (e). plaintiff(s) lives in this district.

PARTIES

5. Plaintiff(s) owns skilled-nursing-home providers incorporated in the states of Illinois and Iowa. The mission of the

All-American Care facilities is to provide skilled-nursing-home services to individuals who require care following the guidelines of Medicare and Medicaid.

6. Plaintiff(s) All-American Restorative Care corporations owners, whose principal place of business is Muscatine and Washington, Iowa, has provided skilled-nursing facility services to individuals who require care following the instructions issued by the federal court pursuant *to Fox v Bowen* Ct. 1986 (ordering HHS/CMS to cease and desist applying arbitrary and capricious rules of thumb) and *Jimmo v. Sebelius*, No. 11-cv-17, D.VT (ordering HHS/CMS to cease and desist imposing an arbitrary and capricious improvement standard).

Legal Standard—Application for Temporary Restraining Order

7. The purpose of a temporary restraining order is to "preserve the status quo and prevent irreparable harm just so long as is necessary to hold a hearing, and no longer" *Granny Goose Food, Inc. v. Bhd. of Teamsters & Auto Truck Drivers*, 415 U.S. 423, 439 (1974). Any temporary restraining order, therefore, is a temporary measure to protect rights until a hearing can be held. There are four prerequisites for the extraordinary relief of a temporary restraining order or preliminary injunction. To prevail, a plaintiff must demonstrate: (i) a substantial likelihood of success on the merits; (ii) a substantial threat of immediate and irreparable harm for which it has no adequate remedy at law; (iii) that greater injury will result from denying the temporary restraining order than from its being granted; and (iv) that a temporary restraining order will not disserve the public interest. *Clark v. Prichard*, 812 F.2d 991, 993 (5th Cir. 1987); *Canal Authority v. Callaway*, 489 F.2d 567, 572 (5th Cir. 1974) (*en banc*). The party seeking such relief must satisfy a cumulative burden of proving each of the four elements enumerated before a temporary restraining order or preliminary injunction can be granted. *Mississippi Power and Light Co. v. United Gas Pipeline*, 760 F.2d 618, 621 (5th

Cir. 1985); *Clark*, 812 F.2d at 993. Otherwise stated, if a party fails to meet *any* of the four requirements, the court cannot grant the temporary restraining order or preliminary injunction.

FACTS

Defendants Violations of the Rule of Law and Administrative Procedure Act

1. Arbitrary and capricious issuance of 2567's and 4972's by the defendants alleging actual harm with severity code G resulting in civil money penalties on numerous occasions posted on the Internet and picked up by the media as factual while the allegations were being appealed and not yet adjudicated and used to smear the plaintiff's reputation and destroy the referral process for acquiring admissions.
2. Defendants arbitrarily and capriciously tying the G violations to the prior provider and trebling the civil money penalties.
3. Defendants triggering a designation as a "special focus" facility requiring punitive exposure to repetitive surveys with the threat of decertification and closure.
4. Arbitrary and capricious revisits by the defendants with resulting allegations and fines resulting in a hold on admissions for five of twelve months of operations causing $1 million in loss of business.
5. Devious and harmful statements and action by the defendants regarding a sexual abuse claim by a patient who was obviously incompetent to make such a claim causing irreparable financial and damaging harm to the defendant owner(s) by posting the allegation, without investigation, on the Internet.
6. Imposition of a conditional license by the defendants requiring compliance upon revisit or revocation of license and closure.
7. A dissident surveyor taking original documents from the facility relating to a patient confidential medical record and not returning them, thereby violating the Privacy and Confidentiality Act (HIPPA) with the defendants ignoring the claim.

8. An RN surveyor alleged that a patient was choking and sat by doing nothing while writing up a deficiency because a nurse was not instantly available to assist a CNA responding to the incident.
9. Requiring that all allegations of patient injury or abuse be self-reported to the defendants regardless of the findings of the provider, thereby violating the Fifth Amendment right to due process of law of having the right to not incriminate oneself and have the right to defend oneself.
10. Defendant's failure to timely issue a decision on the administrative hearing on the first allegations for over a year and a half.

The doctrine of the rule of law dictates that government must be conducted according to law.

Dicey identified three essential elements of the Constitution that were indicative of the rule of law:

- Absence of equality before the law;
- The Constitution is a result of the ordinary law of the land.

Administrative Procedures Act

Standard of judicial review

The APA requires that in order to set aside agency action not subject to formal trial-like procedures, the court must conclude that the regulation is "arbitrary and capricious, an abuse of discretion, or otherwise not in accordance with the law." However, Congress may further limit the scope of judicial review of agency actions by including such language in the organic statute. To set aside formal rulemaking or formal adjudication whose procedures are trial-like (*see* APA, 5 U.S.C 556 - 557), a different standard of review allows courts to question agency action more strongly. For these more formal actions, agency decisions must be supported by "substantial evidence" after the court reads the "whole record," which can be thousands of pages long.

Unlike arbitrary and capricious review, substantial evidence review gives the courts leeway to consider whether an agency's factual and policy determinations were warranted in light of all the information before the agency at the time of decision. Accordingly, arbitrary and capricious review is understood to be more deferential to agencies than substantial evidence review. Arbitrary and capricious review allows agency decisions to stand as long as an agency can give a reasonable explanation for its decision based on the information it had at the time. In contrast, the courts tend to look much harder at decisions resulting from trial-like procedures because those agency procedures resemble actual trial-court procedures, but the Article III of the Constitution reserves the judicial powers for actual courts. Accordingly, courts are strict under the substantial evidence standard when agencies acts like courts because being strict gives courts final say, preventing agencies from using too much judicial power in violation of separation of powers.

The separation of powers doctrine is less of an issue with rulemaking not subject to trial-like procedures. Such rulemaking gives agencies a lot more leeway in court because it is much more like the legislative process reserved for Congress in Article II. Courts' main role here is ensuring agency rules line up with the Constitution and with agency's statutory commands from Congress. Even if a court finds a rule very unwise, it will stand as long as it is not "arbitrary and capricious, an abuse of discretion, or otherwise not in accordance with the law."

Informal Dispute Resolution

We challenge the legality of the IDR process as arbitrary and capricious for the following reasons:

1. Methods are arbitrary and capricious, as explained in our position paper.
2. Fines and penalties are arbitrary and capricious, as explained in our position paper.

3. Ex post facto application of fines based on a survey of a former operator is arbitrary and capricious, as explained in our position paper.
4. Narrowing the constitutional rights of the provider to present its case is arbitrary and capricious, as explained in our position paper.
5. Denying the patients of their constitutional rights to due process of law by imposing punitive damages and penalties that affect their right to privacy and ongoing quality of care, as explained in our position paper.
6. Denying the provider their constitutional right to due process of law by using private information against them in a regulatory process, as explained in our position paper.
7. Any retaliation due to this presentation and position paper will be challenged in the court of law.

February 29, 2012—Arbitrary and Capricious Application of the Rule of Law and Administrative Procedure Act Protecting the Provider's Right to Due Process of Law

All-American Care of Washington requests, as provided by 42 CFR 488.331, an opportunity to refute cited deficiencies at All-American Care of Washington dated February 24, 2012, requiring a plan of correction by March 10, 2012.

On January 25, 26, 30, 31 and February 6 and 7, 2012, a complaint investigation of complaint no. 37483-C and 37531-C was conducted at your facility by Robert Reck, RN, to determine if your facility was in compliance with State licensure and federal participation requirements for long-term care facilities participating in the Medicare and/or Medicaid programs. This survey found the most serious deficiencies in your facility to be:

Scope and severity isolated deficiencies that constitute actual harm that is not immediate jeopardy, whereby significant corrections were required (G); $15,000 fine with $300 per day for noncompliance.

Inadequate nursing supervision. Federal Regulation 483.25(h)(2); State Rule 58.28(3)e, 58.20(2), and 58.20(4)b.

Substantiated.

Based on observation, record review, and two staff interviews, the facility failed to provide adequate supervision and assistive devices for residents at risk for falls. Record review of three sampled residents determined at risk for falls found the facility failed to implement interventions and provide supervision to keep residents safe.

Incontinence care. Federal Regulation 483.25(a)(3); State Rule 58.19(1)j(3).

Substantiated.

Based on observation, record review, and three staff interviews, the facility failed to provide necessary services (incontinency care, bathing) to maintain the personal hygiene of residents unable to carry out the activity independently. Two staff interviewed indicated they have come to work the day shift on the CCDI unit and found residents urine-soaked, sometimes having with multiple bed pads. Observation of facility video on an overnight shift on the CCDI unit found staff failed to enter resident's rooms to check for incontinence in excess of two hours. In an interview, the DON indicated residents on the overnight shift are to be checked for incontinence every two hours and provided incontinence care as needed. Record review also found residents not receiving routine bathing, sometimes not receiving a bath in excess of nine days.

General IDR Information

Facilities may not use the IDR process to delay the formal imposition of remedies or to challenge any other aspect of the survey process, including the following:

- Scope and severity assessments of deficiencies (with the exception of scope and severity assessments that constitute substandard quality of care or immediate jeopardy);

This is a formal request of IDR due to unreported facts and circumstances:

Allegation of substandard care with G level severity warrants further factual information than has been presented and used to establish punitive fines and hold on paying for new admissions. To refute the findings we submit the following underlying circumstances and request that the 2567 be rescinded and resubmitted based on the following:

1. Verbal testimony and facts not reported by Surveyor
2. Documented bathing and staffing schedules not reported
3. Misinterpretation of video records (tampered with 5 clips into 2) to support an allegation that staff did nothing for 48 minutes when in fact testimony proves they were told to leave her on the floor based on her coping with violent behavior without knowing she had fallen no major injury just a bump, no blood from a laceration she received earlier by banging her head on the door frame of her room, no harm when it was discovered on the video that she had fallen out of the view of the one CNA on duty who was told by the Director of Nursing to not approach her until the second aide came on duty which she did while, per her testimony, asking the patient if she was alright who responded yes she was alright. When they did approach her with the additional aide and a nurse, not knowing that she had fallen, assessed her condition according to the nurse, got her up and took her to her room, later finding the 1½ inch laceration with scabbing. The patient was on Coumadin blood thinner so she would have bled all over the floor if she had done it with the fall. There was no bleeding and a small bump next to an inch and a quarter laceration that had scabbing from a previous episode of the patient banging her head against the door frame of her room. So what we really have here is a behavior issue not substandard care.
4. Rob Reck's testimony in the ALJ appeal hearing was filled with I don't knows and distortions of the truth.

5. In-admittance of video review due to HIPPA confidentiality and Quality Assurance restrictions
6. Lack of understanding regarding what the owners are doing at the facility and 2½ months into the turnaround is the basis for a collaborative effort to fix an undesirable situation
7. An Administrative Law Judge decision that is still pending after 1½ years of punishment by the defendants.

Factual concerns and examples regarding the defendant's punitive approach to compliance and complaint surveys as submitted to Rod Roberts, director of the Department of Inspections and Appeals, with copies to the governor of Iowa asking for relief that furthered the retaliation against our businesses. After meeting with the governor and Mr. Roberts in July and August of 2011 and submitting white papers on reinforcement surveys versus punitive surveys and recommending an outcome-based reimbursement program, the retaliation began and is intended to put us out of business and shut me up.

1. *Background of factual unacceptable operating history of prior ownerships.* My family purchased the Washington Facility October 12, 2011 (after purchasing a facility by the same builder in Muscatine in September 2009). The prior operators in both facilities had owned them for many years and had allowed them to decline, become an eye sore, and become an example of poorly managed patient care. Our reputation and success in Muscatine is demonstrated by our survey history; there it speaks for our commitment to changing the view each community has about long-term care. Unfortunately for us, in March 2011, while operating under the prior ownership, Washington was surveyed and found to have a number of deficiencies, resulting in a finding of a class I violation as a result of multiple lesser violations. A fine of $6,500 was imposed for those deficiencies but was reduced by 35 percent in lieu of an appeal. Their problems were well known, and even yet, they were allowed to continue operating at a substandard level.

As is the case with most facilities, when we purchased the facilities, we assumed the provider number of the prior operator. We understand the department and CMS's position is that with respect to assuming the provider number of the prior operator, the new provider assumes certain contingent liabilities associated with that provider number and assumes the prior provider's operating history. The alternative is to apply for a new provider number. Unfortunately, the process of applying for a new provider number is very involved and results in a lengthy delay in the issuance of the provider number, causing a facility considerable cash-flow shortfall. As a result, most providers, particularly smaller independent owners, assume the provider number of the prior operator as a matter of financial necessity. However, this is not considered in the department's approach to making a transition. The defendants want way more than they were getting from the prior owner and make it clear in their conduct and arbitrary interpretation of the rules and regulations.

For example, the defendants conducted a complaint survey at Washington in January and February of 2012, 2½ short months after we assumed ownership of the facility. The complaint survey resulted in alleged deficiencies that included two class I violations. The proposed penalties, which are currently under appeal, involved treble fines. CMS also imposed a denial of payment for new admissions (DPNA) prior to us exhausting our appeal rights. This cost us at least twelve new admissions. Though the State citation did not provide reference to the prior violation giving rise to the treble fine, it appeared to be on the basis that the class I violation was a subsequent or second class I violation and the department concluded it was the same class I violation as a prior class I violation for which a fine was assessed, which occurred during a twelve-month period. The actual elapsed time of 11½ months enabled the defendants to impose the most punitive penalties during the three months it took to make a revisit that was passed with zero deficiencies.

Certainly, the timing of the complaint survey was difficult, as we had not been operating the facility for very long, and it was and continues to be a challenge to change the prior practices and issues associated with Washington prior to our ownership. We believe that the imposition of the treble fines was unjustified in light of these facts and the severity assigned to that violation, and the citation does not provide specific information concerning the alleged repeated violations. Considering the surrounding facts submitted during the survey and subsequent IDR, this treatment is consistent with what should have happened to the previous provider, not us. The previous owner allowed the facility to deteriorate. There were odors, continual flooding in the parking lot, 160 florescent bulbs an eighty-six ballasts burned out contributing to a dark and dreary environment, and a staff that ultimately had to be replaced. According to community leaders, families, and referral agencies, we were miracle workers.

2. *Good faith capital and operating investment in facilities.* My family has invested over $500,000 in capital improvements and upgraded staffing and the quality of the food in each facility. We have also worked on getting family involvement in each of the facilities for which the communities appreciate and will testify to the commitment to our mission (to improve the quality of life for the elderly and disabled). This may not be unique to us as independent owners; however, the significant capital contribution and our performance prior to the implementation of all the surveys and measures by the department were resulting in higher census and significant improvements to patient care with more of our patients going back home. It takes a great deal of time and money to improve a poorly functioning facility, and we have continued to invest that time and money.

Again, I am not suggesting that the department should not survey or inspect facilities; however, I am suggesting that in the case of a new operator who has demonstrable evidence of improved care and resident and family satisfaction, the department should collaborate with the facility and the owner/operator to further improve the care and make necessary corrections, rather than a purely punitive approach. At this stage, we are spending significant sums of borrowed money defending our appeal rights just to stay in business, but that does not come close to our loss of business and DIA staff's flagrant disregard of the intent of administrative procedures prior and subsequent to assessing punitive severity levels to warrant civil money penalties and special-focus status.

3. *Egregious result of the January/February 2012 complaint survey at Washington.* The survey that started this destructive process was a survey conducted by the defendant Robert Reck in January and February of 2012, for a complaint not relevant to your staff's final very subjective and arbitrary findings. This was the survey that was conducted approximately a month prior to the end of the twelve-month period from the last standard survey, which was March of 2011, under the prior owner's watch. Mr. Reck relied in

large part during the survey on review of the Washington facility's security camera footage given to him in good-faith effort to show the circumstances surrounding that particular behavioral-problem patient in our special-care unit. We provided the video to prove that the surrounding circumstances supported our staff's actions.

As a part of our quality-control procedures and keeping our staff accountable, we installed this video security system at the facilities. The camera was used by each facility for quality-assurance activities and follow-up on complaints. During the survey process, the defendant requested copies of the video footage, and Washington, in good faith, complied with those requests. However, the defendant Mr. Reck took the videos out of the context of the facts, testimony by staff and documentation provided him, and relied purely on the tampered video footage to conduct a large portion of his review. Obviously, the video footage had limitations and was not intended for the purpose for which Mr. Reck used it.

For example, the defendant Mr. Reck reviewed the video with respect to an incident involving a psych patient who, we discovered after the incident, had fallen. Though the patient was not seriously injured, he used this video to distort the facts and almost exclusively to construct his version of the incident. Not only did he use the video for his arbitrary and capricious interpretation of the factual basis for the deficiency, he disregarded the context of the situation (the patient had been banging her head on the wall earlier in the day) and based the tag on his interpretation of what occurred after she had fallen. The allegation is that the staff left the resident completely unattended for forty-eight minutes. That simply is not true. We presented facts that the resident had a history of lying on the floor in her closet, in her room, and in the hall as a typical coping behavior, that she had been aggressive with the staff on the day in question, so the staff had been instructed to approach her in pairs, and that at the time of the incident, there was no indication that she had fallen or was injured. Be that as it may, my staff did check with her several times to confirm she was OK. Each and every time the staff asked, she said she was okay, so the staff did not approach her, reasonably concluding she was lying on the floor, consistent with her behavioral coping patterns leading up to the incident. We presented testimony concerning these facts in the IDR process and presented those facts again in the formal appeal. The testimonies were discredited as not sufficiently supported by written documentation.

The defendant Mr. Reck also used the video to determine whether or not the staff was giving appropriate continence care. Specifically, with respect to the incontinence care, the only observation of the care or alleged lack of care was observation of the facility's video. As can be seen, the video has significant limitations, because there is not a camera in every resident's room and the distances are distorted. Kip Rhoads, as the security system technician, testified that the five video clips did not record all movement and demonstrated that fact at the hearing. The video evidence must be impeached as the original five clips were reduced to two by the defendant and CMS' attorney to only show the elapsed time of forty-eight minutes. It is absolutely unclear to us how he or the defendants could determine such a punitive result given solely on the basis of video footage that doesn't even show the care provided in resident rooms or the context of the events that led up to the fall and the circumstances that existed before and after the fall without considering the testimony of our staff and the surrounding circumstances that led up to the incident. The defendant Mr. Reck did not, however, use the video to review other allegations after honing in on the forty-eight-minute allegation.

We then were treated with disrespect by the defendant, compliance officer, and hearings officer during the IDR hearing, where our witnesses were ignored and our factual presentation rejected, which, in fact, proved that it was a documentation tag, not a substandard care tag. This false conclusion has resulted in punitive damages and our ALJ appeal being put off over a year since the incident. It has also caused over $100,000 in legal fees and loss of business due to the facts never being reported or disclosed on the department's and CMS's websites and the impact of those alleged violations being reported in the newspapers and in the media.

4. *Inappropriate special focus facility designation; survey conducted June 2012.* To add harm to injury, the surveys the defendants have now designated and published Washington as a special-focus facility (one of four in the state of Iowa targeted by CMS as substandard care providers). As a result, Washington is now subjected to more frequent surveys. This designation cannot be appealed, and we have never received specific information concerning the calculation of

the underlying basis for the designation of the special-focus facility status. We have also not received any response with respect to which surveys were included for the purposes of the special-focus-facility designation. We have requested this information from the defendants who gave us the name of a gentleman at CMS. This gentleman has not responded, and that designation occurred in June 2012. Not long after the special-focus-facility designation, the department came in and conducted a revisit survey dated June 2012. We then had our annual survey a week later and were cleared with desk review. We then had the six-month survey that resulted in no significant deficiencies. However, the six-month survey was not counted by the department for purposes of demonstrating progress with the special-focus-facility requirements. We have not yet received a satisfactory explanation as to why that survey is not counted since it only resulted in eight tags of D and E severity levels. It is puzzling why the department uses these tactics to justify such treatment for a new provider in Washington and an effective provider in Muscatine.

5. *Lack of good-faith communications from department staff.* Recently, while the defendant surveyors were in the Washington building, my son, Kip Rhoads, and the administrator, Marty Wills, called the defendant Mindyla White, in good faith, to inquire about an issue with a resident who had been engaging in a number of hallucinations, fantasies, and bad behaviors. The behaviors had escalated to the point that we believed we needed to obtain additional guidance from the department on how to handle this matter. The communication was made in October via telephone call to the defendant Ms. White and involved a description of the circumstances, with the resident's family in the room and listening to the telephone call. The communication included a description of the resident making statements concerning an alleged sexual relationship she believed she was having with Kip Rhoads (the owner) and a resulting pregnancy. All of which was easily discounted based on the patient's age and physical condition.

In good faith, the information concerning the resident's erratic psychotic behaviors were explained to the defendant Ms. White over the telephone together without plan of care. The defendant Ms. White assured Kip and Marty that issues like this were not as uncommon as we might think, and she indicated they would not need to investigate the matter. She told Kip and Marty to pull all the information together and submit a self-report and that the defendant would hold on to for reference if anything else occurred in the future. Approximately ten pages of signed affidavits were presented to the department office that proved beyond a doubt that there was no such abuse. Again, the patient's family members were in the room and were apologizing, stating that she had made statements in the past about being pregnant from other men that she had never been with. The family was extremely embarrassed and apologetic concerning this matter.

Later that month in October 2012 on the self-report website, there was an indication that the allegation being made by the resident was going to be investigated. However, on November 2, 2011, the defendant Ms. White called the Washington facility and said that the department was not going to investigate the allegations with respect to this particular resident, but then used it in the 2567, which was posted on the self-report website as a so-called another example of the alleged failure to follow the facility's abuse policy for an unrelated outstanding complaint survey visit in which an allegation of abuse concerning a particular CNA had occurred. At the time that the conversation with the defendant Ms. White in November occurred, that complaint survey had not yet been completed. We asked the defendant, Ms. White, what that would mean concerning the scope and severity levels on the outstanding survey, and she refused to comment.

Again, our concern was that this allegation was reported, in good faith, to the department to the defendant Ms. White, who told us that there was nothing to be concerned about. She later changed her position, and we believe this was inappropriate. They then posted this egregious interpretation on the website and we asked our attorney, Heather Campbell, to contact the department's general counsel, Deborah Svec-Carstens. Not only were we concerned about this matter being made public without any on-site investigation, but we felt it was written in such a way to defame the "owner" alleged to have committed the sexual abuse. It certainly appears that such misrepresentations are an intentional attempt to punish us for appeals and our attempts to get fair and legal treatment under due process of law.

When we inquired as to why the circumstances surrounding the allegations would be included on an outstanding complaint survey after the defendant Ms. White had advised us that there was nothing to be concerned about, the defendants' Ms. Svec-Carstens responded to our attorney that according to the defendant Ms. White, the allegations when the self-report was made were different than what were described to her via the telephone. Again, we believe that when we call the department and receive information, we should be able to rely on that information. If the defendant Ms. White does not want to comment on the issue in the first place, the she should say so. However, by giving us a specific response, we believed that we are entitled to rely on that response. It is this type of bad-faith treatment that turns this into the appearance of retaliation and intentional publication of an incrimination that should result in defamation charges against the department. (This defamatory allegation still resides on the public-access defendants' website as factual.)

There have also been circumstances in which the defendant surveyors have represented, during the exits, that they have made no particular findings or concerns with respect to a particular issue, and following that conversation, the allegations or questions show up on the 2567 as G level violations, thereby justifying a $5,000 fine. Specifically, during the exit interview for Muscatine for the survey conducted in August to September, the surveyor told the staff during the exit that she had no concerns related to the resident who was identified as resident no. 2. Yet when we received the 2567, the department included resident no. 2 as one of the two residents for which the defendants alleged deficiencies. The result was a $5,000 fine and a scope and a tag with a G scope and severity. We are again forced to endure the time and cost of an IDR process that gives the provider few, if any, rights to due process and objective decisions. Our appeal was rejected as not properly documented, so the allegation of substandard care is really a documentation deficiency that does not warrant a G level of severity established arbitrarily by the defendant compliance officer who never personally investigated the incident.

For the Washington compliant survey that is under appeal, one of the surveyor's findings related to equipment. However, when we received the 2567 and State citation, the equipment deficiency had been changed by the defendants to support an accident/supervision tag. The defendant's position is that the supervisory staff can change the 2567 and/or change the categories of the alleged deficiencies; however, those supervisors are not frontline employees who are in the building inspecting and surveying. The supervisory staff should defer to the observations and findings of the inspectors and surveyors that they put in the buildings.

6. *Unprofessional and intimidating conduct of the surveyors during investigation of complaint survey related to alleged abuse.* In addition to the other issues, we have significant concerns related to the conduct of the surveyors during a complaint survey and related allegations of patient abuse. No fewer than nine staff came to us and told us that the surveyors were leading them to only two conclusions: we as managers were guilty by intent or by intimidation of our staff to not report abuse. (In our Muscatine facility during a complaint survey, seven former terminated-for-cause employees were interviewed and quoted in the survey notes to obtain derogatory statements against the owners.) This is not only subjective, arbitrary, and capricious but damaging to us as operators who are having to change a negative culture into a facility that far exceeds the current minimum standards and, in our opinion, provides quality of life as well as complying with DIA's narrow interpretation of quality of care.

7. *Factual inaccuracies on 2567s after provision of information to the contrary.* There have been a number of occasions in which surveyors have provided information with respect to their findings in an exit interview for which we have been able to provide specific information prior to the surveyor leaving the building. For example, in a recent case involving an alleged failure to notify a physician, prior to the surveyor leaving the building, we provided the surveyor with a copy of a document that showed a date and time stamp for a fax notifying the physician of the incident in question. However, when the 2567 was issued, the allegation with respect to failing to notify that physician was on the 2567.

In addition, there are other factual inaccuracies, such as an allegation of a patient coughing in the dining room that was exaggerated into a choking incident by an RN surveyor that made no attempt to help the patient, or the CNA trying to get help. Another was report of an injury of unknown origin that the surveyor concluded was a reportable injury resulting in an abuse/dignity allegation that the cause of the bruising was a result of a gown too tight on the shoulder and that was substantiated as the origin of the injury by the DON and the physician. This is just another example of a completely arbitrary interpretation of the intent of the adult-abuse regulations when it comes to behavioral and troubled geriatric-psychiatric patients that need professional help and can't get it even in a nursing home.

It is our experience with the defendants that they are completely misinterpreting the intent of the regulations and turn what are aberrant behaviors into a violation even though it infringes on our right to manage that behavior and the patients' right to skilled care. Another incident occurred where a patient hit another in our behavior unit, and your surveyors capriciously told us that we should not admit them if it is anticipated that they might harm another resident, or tell us we are working a staff person too many hours trying to justify their interpretation of an alleged violation of a patient incident that clearly did not happen. It just goes on and on as the defendants' interpretation of abuse when it comes down to a very complex care patient. To continue to second-guess on every incident discourages us from taking complex cases, especially when they are not from the Washington area, though no one will take them and they have nowhere else to go.

8. *Governor Branstad and DIA presented with white papers concerning these matters prior to December 2011 complaint survey.* In July and August of 2011, in good faith, I attempted to suggest a better way of conducting the surveys, presented in my book on our past experiences and suggested positive improvements in the survey process and ideas on payment for performance in place of the current punitive enforcement approach to apparently justify civil money penalties. Ironically, after this, we were put through the very process that is damaging the capabilities of the small independent operators to survive this punitive approach to regulatory interpretation of due process of law that takes, in my opinion, the pressure off the State's ineffective management of the Medicaid program.

9. On September 14, 2013, the Department of Inspections and Appeals conducted a complaint survey and alleged that All-American Care should have performed CPR on a dead man. The allegation related to dependent-adult abuse is theorizing that Richard T. was still alive when the nurses decided not to perform CPR and they

caused his death. There is no proof that Mr. Richard T's clinical death was reversible. The tag and resulting IJ and civil penalties allege patient abuse, even to the extent of requiring the abuser to be separated from the abused patient who was clearly dead. Also, we have since been ordered by a directive from DIA to report the nurses to the nursing board for punishment. There is no evidence to support this theory. This resulted in CMS and DIA fabricating an immediate-jeopardy violation carrying with it a conditional license (the fourth freeze on admissions in twenty-six months resulting in eight months of business not being allowed to admit patients), $48,000 in federal fines, and $30,000 in state fines and continued targeting under the special-focus designation imposed twenty-four months ago. We are appealing the allegations based on medical protocol and the facts of the incident.

1. Per CMS ref: S&C 14-01-NH to State Survey Agency directors CPR for nursing homes. Background regarding American Heart Association (AHA), their guidelines deal with the reversal of clinical death since brain death begins four to six minutes following cardiac arrest if CPR is not administered during that time. AHA encourages potential rescuers to initiate CPR unless: (1) a valid DNR order is in place; (2) obvious signs of clinical death (e.g. rigor mortis, dependent lividity, or decomposition); or (3) initiating CPR could cause injury or peril to the patient or rescuer.
2. Reversal of clinical death: Per Dr. Robin Plattenberger, medical examiner, regarding death of Richard T. on 6/2/2013, "According to my investigation, the deceased was in rigor mortis, body cyanotic, and had passed body fluids. The initiation of code not warranted."

This proves our allegation of retaliation or tactic to show us that we do not have any legal rights to due process or the right to improve the quality of life without DIA staff's narrow and arbitrary and capricious interpretation of what is, in fact, quality. How in the world does the governor and HHS/CMS/DIA conclude that negative enforcement will accomplish a positive result that can arbitrarily continue to put well-meaning, more effective small independent owners out of business for the sake of encouraging larger chains to come into Iowa and again gobble up the little guys? I question the intent of the State when it deprives us the very resources that will save Medicaid money by using the Medicare benefits for restoring patients back to the community.

CLAIM

(Declaratory Relief)

1. Plaintiffs repeat and re-allege the foregoing paragraphs as if fully set forth herein.
2. There is an actual controversy between the parties.
3. Plaintiff has received denials for payment due to the defendants' arbitrary and capricious act without explanations as to the reason for denials in accordance with the requirements and the laws set forth in the foregoing paragraphs that the defendants must follow in their determinations.
4. The defendants have caused and imposed three months of admission hold on the Washington facility during the last seven months of our fiscal year ended 12/31/2012 and two months of the first six months o the current year while appeals were being adjudicated causing irreparable harm to the owners, staff, patients, and families causing insurmountable operating losses ($967,000) due to the decline in census from sixty to forty-one during the punitive remedies, legal fees exceeding a $100,000, loss of referral agency use of the provider, causing the provider to seek protection of the courts under chapter 11 of the bankruptcy law.
5. The defendants create severity codes for establishing penalties that enable the imposition of civil money fines then allows for a 35 percent discount (bribe) if the provider agrees not to appeal.
6. The defendants require that the provider copy all the related records and then use them off site to arbitrarily and capriciously create the severity codes for assessing fines and penalties without review or contradiction by the provider who

is led to believe there is no problem, then upon review by the defendants Des Moines staff, they become finable offenses (and in a recent incident, the surveyor took original medical records out of the facility, violating the HIPPA act, and to date, they have not been returned). This is a finable act of $20,000 to $50,000 that DIA is responsible for.

PRAYER FOR RELIEF

WHEREFORE, Plaintiffs, the All-American Care, et al., herby demand judgment as follows:

1. A declaration that the defendants are violating the provisions of the Administrative Procedure Act in the use of "arbitrary and capricious rules in conducting its annual complaint and revisit surveys" and/or use of the informal dispute resolution (IDR) process in denying appeals and claims of punitive treatment of the providers (citations: In *Beechwood v. State of New York*, D. NY, 2012, directed the State to pay the former owner of a Rochester nursing home $25 million. The payment is part of a federal court settlement, after jurors found state health officials improperly retaliated against the owner of the facility in shutting the place down more than a decade ago).
2. A declaration that HHS/CMS/DIA cease and desist not taking into consideration the period of ownership for making improvements and changes in the quality of care.
3. A declaration that the defendants cease and desist using punishment in the media, Internet, to discredit and destroy provider reputations, defame owners, and exert business losses through civil money penalties, hold on admissions and threats to providers who disagree with their gestapo tactics resulting in loss of business, potential bankruptcy filings, and damaging the provider-patient relationship to protect the patients' civil right to care.
4. A declaration that the defendants cease and desist creating allegations through interviewing dissident former employees, using bullying tactics in interviewing current staff, using security videos to incriminate and destroy the intent of such quality-control devices and alleging to newspaper journalists

violations for intentional incrimination (Mr. Kauffman at the Des Moines *Register*) that do not exist.
5. A declaration that the defendants be stopped from making any further postings on the Internet, published allegations for media access, civil money penalty assessments, hold on admissions, issuing special-focus designation by tagging back to a previous owner's provider number, until the provider's due process of law (appeals and court orders) is being exhausted as a prayer for monetary and punitive relief.
6. A declaration that the defendants cease and desist the use of provider or patient incidents as "self-reportable" of alleged violations under the threat of retaliation violating the Fifth Amendment of the constitutional right to not incriminate oneself.
7. A declaration that HHS/CMS/DIA cease and desist the current complaint survey process whereby the complainant does not have to produce their name or connection with the facility nor inform the facility first before reporting the allegation to the defendants who then arrives unannounced with a letter informing the provider they have the right to inspect anything and everything until they find some fall or alleged patient-abuse incident reports lacking their level of arbitrary documentation that they can use against the provider for assessing fines and remedies exerted by CMS in a punitive manner.
8. A declaration that the defendants reimburse the provider for all operating losses, legal fees, loss of business, and punitive damages due to retaliation, defamation of owners, and criminal disregard for the Administrative Procedure Act causing treble damages for monetary and punitive relief.
9. A declaration that the defendants cease and desist the denial of admissions prior to the provider being allowed due process violates the Medicare requirements to give access to beneficiaries that require skilled care.
10. A declaration that the Des Moines Register and its agent, Clark Kauffman, cease and desist printing allegations prior to appeals being adjudicated that damage reputations and defame the provider and its patients who have their civil

rights withheld when they cannot get access to the Medicare and Medicaid services they have the right to receive.

   a. An order granting a temporary restraining order and/or a preliminary injunction should such an order or orders become necessary to protect interest of the plaintiffs or their members.

   b. An order awarding plaintiffs their costs of this action and their reasonable attorney fees.

   c. An award of such other relief in law and equity that this court deems just and proper in the premises.

DAMAGES (Declaratory and Punitive Relief)

1. Personal business losses occurring due to the retaliation of defendants of $670,000 for 2012 and $200,000 for current 2013 due to census decline from sixty at Washington to forty-one now due to the hold on admissions exerted by the defendants.
2. Personal obligation to pay legal fees of $100,000 accrued fighting the defendants' action.
3. Personal irreparable harm and damages due to defendants publishing arbitrary and capricious information on the Internet and in the news media for treble punitive damages individually for retaliation, defamation of owners, and disregard of owner's right to due process of law of $10 million each.
4. Payment of treble punitive damages for the impact this has had on the civil rights of patients to quality of care and quality of life that is being denied when defendants damage the provider's ability to survive financially when the care exceeds the legitimate application of the rule of law and administrative procedures of $90 million.

CHAPTER EIGHT

HOW OUTPUT-BASED HEALTH CARE WINS

PROVIDER BILL OF RIGHTS

In the scheme of things in health care, it seems to me that the small providers are being attacked by the regulators because DIA is not accountable and the most serious problems are left to heap blame on the providers. For example, peri-care (changing diapers in long-term care) is the surveyors' focus when we should be focusing on toileting and prevention of erratic urination. Ninety-nine percent of the caregivers are mothers who have changed diapers for years without all the precautions imposed and used for fines on the smaller nursing homes. Another area of intense focus is on how we pass (put in peoples' mouths) twenty pills a day, sometimes three times a day, right at a prescribed time of day when we should be questioning why anybody over sixty-five should have twenty pills a day (the average in nursing homes is 14.8). In addition, the so-called quality of care minimum standards, devised by the universities and think tanks with government grants, on advocacy for the patients, become the maximums and do not improve quality care or quality of life at all.

The providers are held hostage by the surveyors for these types of regulations, and punitive tactics are used that have destroyed the creativity and initiative of the providers, creating fear factors used to blame the providers and causing a culture of incompetence. Therefore, I am proposing legislation to pass a bill of Provider Rights in order for accountability to be imposed on the regulators who are not concerned about quality of life, just their subjective, arbitrary, and capricious interpretation of institutionalized quality of care without concern for humane quality of life.

Following is the statement of ten provider rights that will improve the providers' performance in a positive and constructive manner versus the existing negative and punitive approach used by DIA to keep the providers afraid to innovate better methods:

1. Surveyors are to explain why they are coming on-site and who has asked them to investigate any complaint. The complaint must have been presented to the provider first and, if not corrected before the surveyor arrives, will be subject to investigation for any patient, family, staff, or former staff complaints. The complainant and a detailed description of the complaint must be identified, and no other issues will be investigated unless covered by a notice of why it is being addressed.
2. Surveyors are to present the concerns they have as they go along and allow the provider time to fix them as they are pointed out. If the solution or correction is not presented while on-site, the surveyor then establishes a tag that will need a plan of correction prepared by the provider and approved by the Department of Inspections and Appeals (DIA). The provider will be allowed twenty days from the date of the 2567 to present a plan of correction, and DIA must approve in ten days. Any referral to CMS for hold on admissions must be deferred until the administrative appeal rights have been exhausted by the provider.
3. The severity established by DIA is to be discussed with the provider by the on-site surveyor before it is established and additional evidence can be submitted before the final level of severity is published. No 2567 shall not be published on the Internet or any other media until all appeals have been adjudicated.
4. The informal dispute resolution (IDR) should be independent of DIA and shall be on the record and the results published for the dissemination to the providers for their edification and use in complying with DIA's interpretations and guidelines.
5. Civil money penalties (fines) shall be established by DIA and CMS after appeals have been adjudicated. Providers are allowed to contest the degree of the penalties in their plan

of correction. If the penalties are harmful to the provider's ability to pay and continue to serve its patients, they would be deferred and be reconsidered in the circumstances as egregious to the care and safety of the patients.
6. No publication will be allowed on the Internet or in news articles until the facts have been adjudicated in the appeal process. Compliance with the Administrative Procedure Act is incumbent on DIA, IDR, Department of Human Services (DHS), and CMS.
7. Any allegation of criminal conduct, sexual or verbal abuse, shall be investigated by the police before being published in the 2567. Defamation of individual or provider character, reputation, and performance is to be discouraged and chargeable as a misdemeanor against DIA personnel.
8. DIA is required by statute to not be arbitrary and capricious in their conduct of their duties and are accountable to governor's office for investigation and resolution. DIA is not allowed to use attack and spread tactics when they investigate allegations and complaints. To expand the survey for the purpose of checking other matters is considered to be outside their authority unless they present justification to the provider in advance of their expanding their investigation.
9. Providers have the right to discharge patients that do not pay their bills or comply with their published policies and procedures. It is the State of Iowa's Department of Human Services (DHS's) responsibility to place its recipients elsewhere if there are unpaid bills, disputes on services, and uncooperative/noncompliant patients.
10. Providers of any size or ownership are to be treated fairly, objectively, and the same in all circumstances with its peers. If not, the violation is considered an allegation of law and must be presented to the State of Iowa attorney general for investigation and resolution. Providers have invested time, hundreds of thousands of dollars, risk their future, committed their reputations in pursuit of quality of care and quality of life. This investment must be honored and taken into consideration to avoid arbitrary use of allegations to hurt providers. The use of intimidation, threats, fear tactics

have not been productive, do not improve outcomes, and destroy provider confidence and willingness to cooperate, finally giving up to large corporate ownership. The small independents (mom-and-pops) are being forced out of business, and the rural communities are going to be deprived of their nursing homes due to operating losses and run-down conditions. (Where are the aging baby boomers going to go for extended restorative care so they can have a quality of life, not just an institutional end of life?)

CHAPTER NINE

MONOPSONY COMMITS FRAUD AND ABUSE

Government Corruption—The Sleeping Giant

EXAMPLE ONE

Written Statement by Sharon Rhoads, who's mother Dorotha White, was killed by the "land of Oz" mentality that permeates government regulators.

Lexington of Lake Zurich knowingly and willfully deprived Dorotha White of the care for which they were being paid that ultimately caused her death on May 16, 2004. Following are excerpts from the Illinois Department of Public Health's inspector Paula Brennan and Public Health's notice of violations:

> On April 25, 2004 Dorotha was found by family to be lethargic, confused and in need of medical attention. Dorotha was transferred to the Emergency Room at family's request and admitted directly from the ER into the ICU with diagnoses of Acute Renal Failure, Congestive Heart Failure, Hypotension and Lethargy. Per interview with Dorotha's primary physician, Dr. Percival Bigol, and Cardiologist Dorotha was severely dehydrated upon admission to ER on April 25, 2004. Dr. Bigol stated that Dorotha had also suffered a Heart Attack prior to admission to the hospital and that her Renal Failure was secondary to the Heart Attack and Dehydration.
>
> Denial of Payment for new admissions effective July 1, 2004 and remedied through the accepted POC.

The facility failed to notify the physician regarding Dorotha's change in physical condition and mental status, high frequency of refusal to take medications and multiple low blood sugar readings. The facility neglected Dorotha and failed to accurately assess and monitor fluid intake did not meet estimated needs, failed to reassess hydration risk after a change in condition was identified, failed to have a hydration plan in place and document alternative attempts to provide fluid, and failed to assess rising Blood Urea Nitrogen (BUN) levels in relation to hydration status. The effective date of the remedy is June 3, 2004. The total amount of the civil money penalty shall be $9,150.

Termination effective December 3, 2004. All imposed remedies will be effective until the facility achieves "substantial compliance" with all federal certification regulations. Before a revisit will be considered, the facility must provide an acceptable POC for all deficiencies documented during the survey at the "B thru L" levels of "Scope and Severity."

Fact: Paula Brennan, Illinois Public Health investigator, found that 118 medications were confirmed to have been missed between February 4, 2004 and April 23, 2004, twenty low blood sugar results between March 1, 2004 and April 4, 2004 resulting in Dorotha suffering hypoglycemia symptoms of anger and increased agitation.

Fact: Hospital records confirm that Dorotha's death on May 16, 2006, was a direct result of the above neglect caused by extreme dehydration and renal failure.

Fact: The physical and emotional abuse of her personal and civil rights to care, lack of competent staff, and willful disregard to her quality of life as resulted from the noncompliance to the following regulations:

1. 42 CFR 483.13 Facility practices—did not follow admission policies and procedures, did not properly manage staff toward safety.

2. 42 CFR 483.15 Quality of life—violated Dorotha's dignity with diapers, nakedness.
3. 42 CFR 483.10 Resident's rights—did not respond to Dorotha's right to competent medical care including lack of care planning and follow-up on acute health needs.
4. 42 CFR 483.25 Quality of care—Disregard to policies and procedure regarding nutrition, hydration, prevention of falls, continence needs, recovery of patient valuables, hearing aids, and eye glasses.
5. 42 CFR 483.75 Administration—lack of professional management of MDS and care plans with no restorative services offered.
6. 42 CFR 483.40 Physician services—nonapproval of psychotropic drug use, order of twenty medications without power-of-attorney approval.
7. Contract with medical director (conflict of interest and self-dealing)—twenty-four Part B claims submitted to Medicare the same day.
8. Failure to follow facility policies and procedures for preventing dehydration, malnutrition, falls, abuse, and injury prevention.
9. Failure to follow facility policies and procedures for notification of use of psychotropic medications, medication administration, blood sugar monitoring, and restorative programming for which the facility was being paid.
10. Failure to report the above to the state of Illinois Public Health Department as required by CFR 483.25.

Fact: Above are the citations taken from Public Health's investigation prior to reducing the allegations to lower violations and assessing Lexington with a watered-down statement of deficiencies of public record that resulted in inconsequential civil money penalties of $3,050 per instance for F157, F224, and F327 or a mere $9,150 for causing Dorotha White's untimely and painful death.

The following facts dictate that the department's abatement of "immediate jeopardy" deficiencies are not supported by the degree of the violations and that a B violation is not representative of the severity of the immediate jeopardy acts, nor the corrective punitive action adequate to hold the management of Lexington accountable for Dorotha White's death:

Fact: Lexington is operated by Royal Management, located in Lombard, Illinois. The Samatas brothers, who are the owners and operators of the Lexington facility in Lake Zurich, are responsible for the above violations and willful disregard for the public-health standards and regulations. In Royal Management's written plan of correction (POC) to the affirmed violations (numbers 4, 6, and 9) stated above, they categorically blame the staff at Lexington and propose to fix it with a few belated in-services.

I contest the State's contention that there is no pervasive "immediate jeopardy" to all Lexington residents and the fact that they did not enforce all of the above stated violations. All were warranted by the following facts that can be confirmed by staff members and other families if subpoenaed in a court action that we are prepared to carry out:

1. Dorotha expired as a result of the neglect, abuse, and substandard care documented by the Department of Public Health in the investigation presented by Paula Brennan, RD (RD meaning registered dietician, not a RN or MD). This proves beyond a doubt that her civil and personal rights to care were violated and the state of Illinois is negligent in allowing Lexington to continue to operate as a licensed skilled-nursing facility as evidenced by the following:
    a. Dorotha was not properly diagnosed by Dr. Bianchi. He claimed she suffered from Alzheimer's disease, which, in fact, was confirmed by her previous doctor, Dr. Bigol, to not be the case. As a result, she was moved to the third-floor locked unit and treated accordingly. Also, with Alzheimer's as the justification, Dr. Bianchi prescribed Haldol, a psychotropic medication on April 24, which further complicated Dortoha's condition without the notification or approval of my power of attorney. He claims he was not informed of her condition but was at Lexington the day before (April 24), administering

Haldol. The next day (April 25), I found my mom in extreme renal failure, unable to swallow and being ignored by the nursing staff. We also received twenty-four Part B bills (for services rendered in February, March, and April) emanating from his so-called lack of involvement in my mother's death.

b. There were 118 medications confirmed to have been missed between 2/10/04 and 4/23/04, twenty low blood sugar results between 3/1/04 and 4/25/04 resulting in Dorotha suffering hypoglycemia symptoms of anger and increased agitation (for which Dr. Bianchi prescribed Haldo to treat). As power of attorney, I was not informed of any of these results or actions. Around the middle of February 2004, the head nurse (Judy) told me that they were withholding mom's medications because she didn't eat enough. I called Dr. Bianchi's office and left a message with the receptionist to have Dr. Bianchi give a standing order at Lexington that mom's medications not be withheld. She assured me he would get the message.

c. On April 25, when we found my mom was near death, she had not been fed, nor could she swallow the food we tried to feed her. Over a period of two months, she had not been taking in enough calories for sustaining her weight or health.

d. The facility's nursing staff was nonresponsive when I approached them on numerous occasions on Mom's weakened and debilitated condition. These are of record through my signing in at the reception desk and complaints registered with social service personnel and nursing staff and administration. I met with facility administration, wrote to the owners, attended care-plan meetings, visited my mother almost every weekend to check on her condition, and found the staff incapable due to shortage in staff.

e. During my mom's stay, I reported the loss of personal belongings, glasses (at least ten times), hearing aids (two destroyed in the laundry), personal clothing lost (on occasion, all her underwear was missing), and lack of dignity by finding her partially nude in bed, with nursing administration stating that it was their policy to put someone incontinent to bed nude so they would not contract bed sores. Many times I found her without her bra, wearing wrong or inappropriate shoes, or with multiple clothing items on her roommate that belonged to Dorotha.

f. Dorotha was put in diapers though the nursing staff indicated that she was not incontinent and put in a wheelchair though she could ambulate without assistance, up to the last week she was at Lexington (I walked her the weekend before April 25 outside the facility).

g. Complete lack of therapeutic or restorative services. I had to insist that she be put in physical therapy after a fall, and there were no restorative services provided though the state Medicaid is paying for them in their daily rate. Dorotha should have been hospitalized for her pneumonia, heart attack, and weakened condition so therapy could be prescribed and carried out as required by the Medicare and Medicaid programs.

2. The staffing was never posted in the lobby as required by public-health regulations, conditions of participation in Medicare and Medicaid. Based on our personal observation, the third floor staffing on weekend, particularly Sundays, was pitifully short (one nurse and two staff CNAs for seventy beds and at least sixty patients on average).

a. The investigation by Public Health did not embrace staffing at all except to spend pages in the statement of violations incriminating a staff person on the second floor who was blamed by administration for their problems and terminated for abusing second-floor residents.

b. In the investigation of the violations, the state did not review, document, or analyze the staffing patterns for the third floor in relation to the requirements for such compliance. The investigation avoids this issue and, without any facts, concludes they could not make a determination of the adequacy or inadequacy of staff then merely passes on this issue in the survey report of violations.

c. Facility administration, based on our expert knowledge of the licensing requirements for the State of Illinois Department of Professional Standards (we are healthcare consultants in the nursing-home business, and my husband is a licensed administrator) was incompetent and nonresponsive to Dorotha's rights to care during her stay and specifically for her medical needs for hospitalization the last week at Lexington.

   i. During the 9½ months Dorotha was there, at least two different administrators, along with new directors of nursing, social services, and floor staff. The staff on the third floor on the weekends mainly consisted of housekeeping staff who were incapable of dealing with Dorotha's needs.

   ii. Complete lack of compliance with the federal resident-assessment instrument (MDS) requirements that care plans are to be prepared and updated as the change in condition warrants. None of these requirements were adequately followed during her 9½ months at Lexington nor in that last week during her obvious critical medical crisis.

d. The charge nurse on duty April 25 when we found my mom was an agency nurse and did not know my mom, nor did she seem to be concerned that I found her hanging in her wheelchair, moaning and crying out for help at the nursing station.

   i. We attempted to feed her. When she could not swallow, we decided to insist on hospitalization.
   Her tongue was swollen, cracked, and bleeding from lack of fluids.

   ii. My husband insisted that we call Dorotha's former attending physician, Dr. Bigol, and get her into Alexian Brothers, not Dr. Bianchi's choice.

   iii. The charge nurse finally, after I threatened to call 911, got Dr. Bianchi to authorize a discharge to Alexian Brothers. The daughter and son-in-law intervened

  and called their personal physician who discharged her to Humana Hospital, where she died ten days later.
 iv. After the paramedics took her to the hospital, the charge nurse falsified the facts in a written nurses' note regarding her version of the discharge. (We provided copies to the investigator who indicated the nurse could not be found for interview.)

This medical malpractice is a complete disregard of Dorotha's health, welfare, and civil rights to care being funded by the state and federal Medicare and Medicaid programs and resulted in my mom's death:

1. For a mere $9,150 in civil money penalties and management blaming *facility staff* and submitting a shallow POC with belated in-services, Lexington is allowed to continue their criminal practices. Facility absentee ownership obviously has been allowed to wiggle out of their responsibilities stated in the conditions of participation that they have committed to in their Medicare and Medicaid contract.
2. We believe that the facts justify decertification of Medicare and Medicaid contracts based on violation of the Medicare conditions of participation and loss of license remedies available to the state of Illinois for willful disregard for the safety and care of Dorotha White, and others, that resulted in her violent and painful death (ten days in ICU and hospice at Alexian Brothers Hospital and another eleven days on hospice at Alden Convalescent Center) causing extreme pain and grief of her family.
3. Our attorneys are pursuing legal remedies based on these facts. We have been notified by at least two other families that have similar experiences at Lexington of Lake Zurich and are willing to testify to the facts they experienced with neglect, abuse, and substandard care by Lexington and Dr. Bianachi.

If the State of Illinois does not choose to reopen this case and apply the lawful remedies available to them, we will take the proper legal action to expose their wanton disregard for the responsibilities accorded them by federal law under the Social Security and Civil Rights Act.

Signed: _____ Date: _____
       Sharon K. hoads, Daughter of Dorotha White

Witness: _____ Date: _____
       Sharon K. White Rhoads: Daughter's Written Statement
       Regarding Dorotha C. White's Death on May 16, 2004

Dorotha C. White's civil, health, and welfare rights were violated by Lexington of Lake Zurich that led to her untimely death on May 16, 2004. In the process, 42 USC 12101 and 1395i-3, 1396r and 42 CFR 483 subpart B, as embodied in the conditions of participation for Medicare and Medicaid certification, were violated by Lexington of Lake Zurich.

Citation of Law:

Under the United States Constitution and federal law, nursing home residents have a right to reasonably safe living conditions, adequate health care, restorative and rehabilitative care services, freedom from unreasonable restraints, and a treatment setting that is the most integrated and appropriate based on individual resident needs. See United States Constitution Amendments I, XIV; *Youngberg v. Romeo,* **457 US 307 (1982);** *Olmstead v. LC,* **527 US 582 (1999). Federal statutes governing the operation of nursing homes and their implementing regulations create similar rights. See, e.g., Americans with Disabilities Act, 42 USC § 12101 et seq. (ADA); Section 504 of the Rehabilitation Act of 1973, 29 USCA § 794 (Section 504); Grants to States for Medical Assistance Programs (Medicaid) 42 USC § 1396r; Health Insurance for Aged and Disabled (Medicare) 42 USC § 1395i-3; 42 CFR § 483 Subpart B.**

The detailed investigative report by Paula Brennan, RD, an investigator for the Illinois Department of Public Health, documented forty-six pages of findings of immediate jeopardy on all counts and

Lexington's admitted need for training of staff on policies and procedures. This documentation proves that Dorotha White's death was a result of level J and G violations, not isolated or limited to Ms. White. In light of the department's questionable reduction of the findings to "potential harm" and based on the investigative findings, we request that an extended survey be conducted by CMS and the US Attorney and that Lexington's Medicare and Medicaid funding be retroactively withheld from May 16, 2004, until the extended survey is complete.

In that survey, further investigation needs to be made of the conflict of interest of Dr. Bianchi, medical director of Lexington and also the attending physician for Ms. White. The report discovered that Dr. Bianchi, who claims he was not informed by Lexington staff of Ms. White's condition, gave her a psychotropic Haldol injection, without family consent, on the twenty-fourth of April, the evening before the family found her near death and had her hospitalized. Dr. Bianchi also signed orders resulting in twenty-four Part B Medicare bills from January through April 2004.

In addition the IDPH, IDR process made an interpretation of the investigative report and reduced it to twenty-four pages of immediate jeopardy and indicated there were no apparent violations of Ms. White's patient rights nor was there a lack of trained staff available for her needs. Strangely, the immediate jeopardy tags were reduced to "potential harm" by IDR and later remanded by CMS to a "harm" level. This resulted in the CMPs being reduced from a potential of $10,000 per day per violation to $3,050 per violation, if Lexington did not choose to appeal. Amazingly, the violations went from level J and G to level A then to B.

But the facts demonstrate that Ms. White's rights "to reasonably safe living conditions, adequate health care, restorative and rehabilitative care services, freedom from unreasonable restraints, and a treatment setting that is the most integrated and appropriate based on individual resident needs" were violated (see citation above). Not only did the investigator find that her rights were violated but that the state of Illinois Public Aid Division is paying Lexington for restorative and rehabilitative services and they are not being provided. We believe the Illinois attorney general and the justice department should be brought in to investigate this matter.

Also, the facts are reported in the investigative report that the Lexington staff was not properly trained, which is Lexington's ownership's position in its plan of correction approved retroactively by IDPH. If this is the case, how could the staffing be adequate to take care of any patient's needs, let alone Ms. White's? We ask that this be investigated more thoroughly during the extended survey by pulling staffing records and determining who, in fact, was on duty during the period of January 2004 to May 31, 2004.

The administrative law judge held that the lack of standing of the family to question CMS or state fines and remedies deprived Sharon Rhoads the right to question the fact that the final assessment of fines and remedies against Lexington were reduced from $2 million to $3,350 with no CMS hold on admissions or fines.

The Rhoads family engaged an attorney and settled a wrongful death case against Lexington and lived to fight again.

ATTORNEY'S RESPONSE: "WHY WOULD WE WANT TO SUE OUR FRIENDS AT THE STATE?"

EXAMPLE TWO

Dear prospective attorney, have you experienced retaliation by CMS/DIA? I badly need help, although Heather Campbell with Fredricks is handling the ALJ appeal. I need a litigator. In the ALJ hearing, it was established that the evidence (security videos) had been tampered with by CMS to make their allegation of nothing being done for a patient on the floor for forty-eight minutes, and Mr. Reck, the surveyor, perjured himself a number of times in his testimony. I have tried to get association help to no avail. Their advice is to turn off the security system and gut it out.

For your information, my wife, son, and I purchased Washington Care Center from Randy Lange October 12, 2011, and completely renovated outside and most of inside at a cost of $500,000 as we had in Muscatine. On December 23, 2011, unknown to anyone, there was a fall in our CCDI unit. Kip Rhoads, my son, had put in security cameras to monitor quality issues that he used to discover that a psych patient had fallen. On January 12, 2012, Rob Reck from DIA arrived on a complaint related to heat and a staff person sleeping in the unit.

Of course, he started with falls, and Marty Wills, the administrator, in good faith, offered up five video clips that showed the patient falling. There was testimony by the staff that they were told by the DON to not approach the patient unless there were two staff persons because she lay on the floor as a coping mechanism and was violent if disturbed. Forty-eight minutes later (as alleged by Rob Reck), the staff slowly approached the patient now knowing she had fallen. There was no blood; the patient was conscious and responded to the nurse who accompanied the two CNAs. In IDR, we presented testimony by the nurse and CNA that they had talked to her before and after the fall from the nursing station, which was only forty feet from where she was lying.

She was assessed by the nurse and returned to her room where they found a bump and a laceration of 1½ inches that had coagulated. The patient was on Coumadin, so the laceration happened earlier when she tore up her room, banged her head on the wall, and pulled on the privacy curtain. There is documentation that she was lying on her closet floor and in the hallway over the previous ten days. Reck assumed that the laceration was caused by the fall, and the G was for substandard care and poor supervision of staff. During a complaint survey after this incident, my son was accused by a demented 350-pound sixty-nine-year-old patient of getting her pregnant. In a panic, he called Myndila White, who indicated not to worry, that he should get statements from the family that in no way could this happen, which he did. They then published the incident in the 2567 on the Internet, using it as example that we had not followed our patient-abuse policies. Reading as if it had really happened and when Heather threatened to sue them for defamation, they changed the word *owner* to *administration*.

This resulted in a double G; tied back to Lange's G, it put us in special focus, fined $18,000, and held our admission for three months, and our appeal is still pending after $70,000 in legal fees. Our census plummeted from sixty to forty-six. We are now at forty-four after having to pass on sixteen referrals from the University of Iowa Hospital. We were smeared on the Internet and by Clark Kauffman in the *Register* and local news media resulting in a fiscal-year loss of $700,000 due to this punishment. We are now on hold again with a conditional license for alleged tags that are trumped up, and DHS and CMS are threatening decertification and shipping the patients out. We have decertified the CCDI and plan to provide bariatric rehab to stimulate census referrals. The University of Iowa has been a positive backer of our willingness to accept difficult cases and have indicated they will fill us up with bariatrics since nursing homes won't take them. Of course, DIA could care less about the human element. During our revisit for the self-reported fall, they claimed we had a wound-care deficiency and forced to bring in Telligen, a consultant to DIA, to coach us on infection control and wound care. We had all three wounds, and Telligen wondered why they had been called in because there were no wound problems.

Why would DIA choose to continue to harass and hurt our patients care, our families, my family, and the community of Washington? Because they can, and in my case, it is intentional since, after having success in Muscatine, I had approached the governor and Rod Roberts about changing the survey process to collaboration instead of punitive tactics and pay for results, not average rent, pills, and diapers. It looks like I pulled on Superman's cape and this is what the Rhoadses get for getting out of line.

Jerry L. Rhoads, CPA, CEO All-American Care Centers

Postscript: After all this, we were put on a conditional license with all admissions forbidden that lasted another two months, so in five of twelve months, we were on admission hold, and we still do not have a decision from the ALJ on the video incident. I have yet to find an attorney that will help us hold DIA to due process of law. As a result of a failed revisit on a fall, we were issued another G violation, fines, and a conditional license depriving us of admitting anyone. —Jerry Rhoads, 9/23/2013

Then in October 2013, Shari Rhoads was goaded into firing Crystal, our dietary manager, and her two daughters for insubordination. Crystal proceeded to write a complaint letter to the State, and they arrived with their digging shoes on. As a result, with help from Crystal, they questioned the death of Richard T. According to the surveyors, the staff should have performed CPR on this dead man. Of course, after much bullying of the CNAs and nurses, they claimed there were no policies and procedures in place for DNR/CPR. This resulted in an IJ, eight days' fines at $6,000 per day, totaling $48,000 plus $30,000 treble damages for the state citations. The family, the medical examiner, the attending physician, and our medical director said it was inappropriate to perform CPR on a man that was obviously expired. Of course, the allegations were false since we did have policies and procedures in place and the staff failed to follow them. As in all other citations, we have appealed. —Jerry Rhoads, 11/23/2013

CHAPTER TEN

ENTERPRISE HEALTH CARE PASSES GO

AND FINDS THE SOLUTION

THE RESTORATIVE MODEL OF CARE

What is the Restorative Model of Care? It is the systematic software program for restoring each patient's functional level. Using our caregiver management system, we assess each person's capability to perform baseline activities of daily living, set outcome goals for improvement, and track their improvement for the following:

1. *Walking* and balancing themselves safely without the fear of falling,
2. *Dressing* themselves from clothing to shoes and socks,
3. *Grooming* themselves facially and hairwise,
4. *Expressing* themselves audibly and understandably,
5. *Bathing* themselves fully and safely,
6. *Moving* themselves in bed to avoid pressure ulcers and breakdown,
7. *Feeding* themselves safely without choking or aspiration,
8. *Taking* medications and going to the doctor regularly if depressed or ill,
9. *Interacting* socially with friends and family,
10. *Asking* for help if feeling ill or weak,
11. *Making* decisions about their daily activities,
12. *Handling* financial affairs reasonably well.

The restorative process is organized and put into action using the caregiver software for assessment, problem definition, program development, and assignment of the interventions to the nursing, therapy, and social services teams for implementation. Time frames are established for each of the outcome goals and progress monitored using deficit scales:

- 4 = total dependence on staff for safe performance
- 3 = extensive assistance of staff for safe performance
- 2 = limited assistance of staff for safe performance
- 1 = supervision only by staff for safe performance
- 0 = totally independent for safe performance

The Caregiver Management Systems Outcome Manager software has the following components:

- Comprehensive assessment instrument linked to medical diagnosis that has 102 triggers for determining the problem list for each patient and the cause of each problem.
- Model restorative programs linked to the problem lists for each discipline (nurses, therapists, nurse aides, restorative aides, social workers, dietician, and discharge planners).
- The models are from the caregiver library of sixteen thousand diagnosis-driven models linked to the physician's diagnosis and the hospital's discharge summary.
- The work assignments are accessed automatically for each patent's assessment and customized to that patient's daily interventions.
- Each problem has a goal for establishing an outcome that is pursued by each discipline (the baseline numerical deficit is set, and the goal is stated numerically, and the progress periodically tracked by the licensed personnel between the numerical deficit and the numerical outcome).
- The staff is assigned their workload and workflow using these outcome plans of care by day, by shift, by intervention using standardized minutes of care, frequencies of the task and duration of the goals. These assignments can be given on computer tablets, and the time absorption and progress can be documented real time.

The Caregiver Survey Manager software has the following components:

- Assigns the State's F-tags and K-tags to staff positions for compliance,
- Uses the QIS standards for care for establishing facility policies and procedures,
- Compliance officer is responsible for holding staff accountable to the state of Iowa's regulatory standards on a daily basis,
- Allows for developing plans of correction on a proactive basis for training the staff on corrective action as we find the problems; we turn problem makers into problem solvers.

The caregiver staffing manager has the following components:

- Staffing levels are generated by the minutes from the patient outcome manager standard time values and tracked using the point-of-service module.
- Staffing behavior is managed using the "I care" program of points assigned based on positive and negative values assigned by the standards of performance set by management. A base point value of twenty is increased or decreased by each staff person's day-to-day performance and use to set pay raises and perks.

What we are doing, using these methods, is discharging over 50 percent of our admissions back into the community. This saves Medicare $250,000 per year per Medicare patient times the twenty-five we discharge to home every year. That is equal to $625,000 per year by keeping them out of the hospital five times and saves Medicaid for the average stay of a Medicaid patient of 328 days. We have over forty that we admit per year, and twenty go home; that saves Medicaid 7,560 days at $125 per day, which is equal to $945,000 each and every year right here in All-American Care of Muscatine. That is a total of $1.75 million saved by restoring them rather than just housing them. At the same time, we have reduced medication usage by 33 percent or 28,105 patient days times average medication costs of $30 per patient day times 33 percent, which is equal to $278,200 saved by getting patients off inappropriate drugs.

All-American Care is the only restorative-care center in Iowa and is demonstrating the effectiveness of managing the quality of life that reduces costs by $2 million per year to Medicare and Medicaid. It proves that quality is cheaper and more effective than pure institutional care. The restorative model is designed for skilled-nursing facilities to replace the medical model that is for hospital critical-care patients and the social model that is for high-functioning residents in assisted and independent living.

The Caregiver Management software is the proprietary system that was developed and programmed by Jerry, Shari, and Kip Rhoads over the last twenty-five years and has been implemented for Medicare programming in over 140 skilled-nursing facilities and increased the discharges back to the community by over forty thousand cases. They now use the system in their All-American Restorative Care Centers.

PART III
"GOTCHA"

CHAPTER ELEVEN
"GOTCHA RULES THE SHOP"

About the Victims and Author

Jerry Rhoads is a CPA and a fellow in the American College of Health Care Administrators. He has written six books on nursing-home accounting and systems and more than one hundred published magazine articles on health-care reimbursement and cost-systems topics.

He is currently president and chief executive officer of All-American Care Centers, Caregiver Management Systems Inc., a management consulting and software firm specializing in long-term care. He created the caregiver charting, staffing, and cost system while running two skilled-nursing facilities and a CCRC.

He wrote the white paper in 1975 on outcome based reimbursement for HCFA that led to MDS and RUGs development. He also sat on the HEW and HHS committees in the 1970s and 1980s that formulated the current RAI linkage to case-mix formulas based on nursing minutes of care.

Jerry was president and chief executive officer of his own CPA firm that began in 1977 and grew into a consulting firm and software development company. Prior to that, he was a partner in two other CPA firms after leaving the Health Care Consulting Division of Arthur Andersen & Co. in 1969. While there, he was assigned to head up the Blue Cross of America project for auditing claims and cost reports as the first fiscal intermediary for the entire country when Medicare and Medicaid legislation was originally passed and implemented. He later was the partner in charge of the Aetna Insurance Company Fiscal Intermediary project for auditing claims and cost reports.

Jerry's War Stories
Jerry Rhoads as a Son

George and Velma Rhoads were my parents. Born in Missouri during the Depression years, they worked all their lives for a comfortable retirement that never came. They were neither particularly healthy nor wealthy. In their later years, chronic maladies took their toll.

George had worked in the factory at Firestone and contacted respiratory problems from asbestos. He had looked forward to being sixty-four so he could get away from the drudgery of work. At the age of eighty-two, he died in a nursing home where he had been for the better part of four years. Prior to going to the nursing home, he had a stroke that impaired his functioning somewhat, but it was the respiratory problems that prevailed. During the time he was in the nursing home, he fractured his ankle and his wrist due to staff-related accidents. At the latter stages of the emphysema, he was put on continuous oxygen. This was the beginning of the end; due to his dependence on a certain saturation rate, during the night he was delirious and was given sedatives to quiet him. Not only was the protocol harmful, but it eventually killed him. At no time did a doctor see him more often than every ninety days. During that time, he received on average five telephone orders for lab tests, medications, and other doctor-ordered tests that led to furthering his demise.

Velma, my mother, had heart problems related to blood thinners that were prescribed for her as she aged. But the real problem was her digestive system. Diverticulitis developed, and she had to have a portion of her colon removed and a colostomy bag inserted. Having been on blood thinners prior to the operation, she had a blood clot during surgery and had a stroke. From that point on, she could not walk, talk, or move her right side. Her mind was still there, but she could not communicate. She followed my father in death at the age of eighty-four, at the same nursing home, as a vegetable. To stop the suffering, she was taken off life support and starved to death over a ten-day period.

On numerous occasions, I voiced concern and unhappiness about the lack of staff and the misuse of my father and mother's Medicare benefits. The care was subpar, there was never any staff available on the weekends, and it was inevitable that their passing would be inhumane.

Jerry Rhoads's Initiatives as an Administrator

At Fox Valley Nursing Center, in Elgin, Illinois, and Carington Living Center in Glendale Heights, Illinois, we set up restorative and psychosocial programs for improving the patients' functioning through the following activities:

- Bowling league using plastic pins and balls
- Fitness trail for exercise
- Resistance training using light weights and pulleys
- Gourmet club on Saturday and Sunday nights
- Sewing club for sale at the annual bazaar
- Knitting club for sale at the annual bazaar
- Card club
- Current events club
- Personal history club
- Newcomers club
- Stroke club
- Respiratory club
- Heart and soul club
- Theater club and karaoke time
- Happy hour

We also had the more functional patients sorting and folding clothes for which they were paid. All females had their hair done once a week and the men once a month. We had a security plan that included a functional patient checking locked doors at night. We had an Ambassador Club that met every Friday for voicing problems that needed to be addressed the next week. A member of the staff participated along with the resident representative, a family member, the administrator, and a volunteer.

The most memorable people that helped me pull facilities out of the gutter were at Carington. Wally was an ambulatory patient that wanted to be helpful, and Irene was the resident council president that wanted to improve the conditions. Both became my friends and helpers in keeping an eye out for problems and being my eyes and ears during the weekends and nights. They were the reporters to the Ambassador Club that fixed physical and staff problems as they were occurring. Initially, they were called Jerry's spies, then they became my ambassadors of goodwill and care. Both these soldiers of fortune died after I left Carington, probably of a broken heart because I gave them hope and a purpose and the successors gave them a warehouse again.

At Fox Valley, a 207-bed skilled-nursing facility, in 1987, the problems manifested themselves in staffing. The staff morale was low and resulted in no-shows and walk-offs. The state surveyors called it Death Valley because of the problems from the past. One Sunday, I received a call at home that the surveyors entered the center at midnight for the stated purpose of doing a focused review of the care and staffing. I personally drove to the nurse aides' houses to pick them up to work that night shift, or we would have been closed. One CNA voiced concern because she had been drinking all day. I had no choice but bring her in and ask her to stay out of the way of the surveyors. Fortunately, I was able to satisfy them with my commitment to make changes immediately. It was shortly thereafter that the infamous snowstorm happened and half the staff came together as teams and ran the place better for three days. From that point on, the staff organized the care in teams and met the patients' needs consistently, and we were awarded the five stars of quality in our next survey. When the facility was sold in 1989, it had 195 patients, thirty-four Medicare cases and was generating over $3.5 million per year in revenue. Prior to the turnaround, the census was 167 with four Medicare cases and $2 million in revenue.

Interestingly, when I got to Fox Valley, then Carington, the staff did not know what the state's quality incentive payment was all about. QUIP, as it was called, paid a bonus of $2 per patient per day if you scored on all their six criteria of quality. The criteria were called stars and focused on environment, care planning, family involvement, patient satisfaction, productive activities, and infection control. So we went from the staff not knowing what a star was to earning all of them in a matter of days at Fox and a matter of weeks at Carington. How is this possible? Well, we went from departments to teams, we went from warehousing to care housing, and the end result was better care at a lower cost: turnover was reduced from 200 percent to less than 20 percent; unapproved absenteeism went away and the disregard for the patients' needs dissolved overnight. More revenue, less cost, better care—what a formula.

At Carington, in 1989, the staff was again initially resistant to change but responded to the plan to focus their time on the patients' needs with time to socialize with the patients as well as prioritize their care. We were initially rejected for certification by the VA due to lack of programming, but later on a follow-up visit, they could not believe the number of programs we had going daily. At that point, the social service staff was conducting thirteen psychosocial programs daily along with rehab nursing and restorative care being provided to those that needed it on a daily basis. It was their opinion that we were better than the flagship called White Hall. Of course, we got their certification and backing. When I got to Carington, the census was 175 out of 206 beds, they had four Medicare patients, and the revenue was around $2.5 million. Twenty-two months later, we had 197 patients with an average Medicare caseload of fifty-five and annualized revenue of $5 million. Not only did we have the highest Medicaid rate in the state, but we had convinced Medicare to raise the daily rate by $75 per day for rehabbing and restoring cases back home.

Jerry Rhoads's Initiatives as a Consultant

In 1979, at the Methodist Retirement Center in Lawrenceville, Illinois, there was no active Medicare program, and the old shelter care building was slated for demolition. I was brought in as a consultant to help the board avoid bankruptcy. We proceeded to devise an action plan that would raise $3 million in tax-exempt bonds for restoring the shelter care building into an assisted-living concept. Thirty beds were certified for Medicare, and a new administrator hired to run the business affairs replacing a Methodist preacher who had let the operation go downhill. Today, the continuing-care concept that was implemented twenty-five years ago is the flagship for long-term care services in Southern Illinois. They have added duplexes, condos, and town houses for the elderly.

In 2003, Christian Homes (an eleven-nursing home chain in Missouri and Arkansas) engaged my firm to capture the Medicare billings that were justified by the use of the Caregiver Management System utilizing the regulatory requirements of *Fox v. Bowen* and *Transmittal 262*. Unbeknownst to that organization, they had been incorrectly instructed by their intermediary that they could not bill for anything except certain procedures specified by the interpretations of CMS (the paying agency for Medicare). Once we got involved in mapping out the care that Medicare was to pay for and supported their billing with this documentation, the revenue streams increased an average of 30 percent per facility. Since the state Medicaid programs were cutting back, this represented an instant life-support correction for all their facilities. To date, the system has justified upward to $8 million more in annual billings less the savings to the Medicaid program of $4 million.

In 2002, Nursing Home Managers (a five-nursing-home chain in Illinois) engaged my firm to capture lost Medicare billings. Over a three-year period, that group was able to stop sending bills to the state of Illinois Medicaid program and generate another $5 million in revenue.

In 2004, we were engaged by Pinnacle Health Care (with thirteen homes in Arkansas and Missouri) to do the same thing and generated over $11 million per year in additional Medicare billings.

In 2004, we were engaged by ABCM Corporation (operator of thirty-one nursing homes in Iowa) to assist them in capturing lost Medicare revenue. To date, they have implemented Caregiver Management System in six of their homes and have successfully improved their Medicare performance by 25 percent.

In 2003, were engaged by HMR Corporation (operator of twenty-five nursing homes in South Carolina) to assist them in capturing lost Medicare revenue in two of their homes.

In 2006, we were engaged by an owner of two skilled-nursing facilities in Iowa. They were in financial difficulty and did not think they could afford us. We finally got ABCM to recommend us, and to date, both have implemented Caregiver Management Systems. In the one home they had no Medicare cases and, in thirty days, improved to fifteen active cases. In the other facility, they went from four to eight the first day of training by bringing patients back on Medicare that had been inappropriately discontinued. At this rate, the two homes will produce $2.3 million more in revenue and can be solvent.

Over the last fifteen years, we have put the system in over 140 facilities in twenty-two different states (a chain of fourteen in Utah; a chain of eleven in Texas, New Mexico, Louisiana, and Oklahoma; a chain of ten in Ohio; a chain of three in Arizona; a not-for-profit group of six CCRCs in Ohio; homes in Nebraska, New York, California, Indiana; thirty-three facilities in Illinois; a chain of eleven in Missouri; a chain of thirteen in Arkansas, etc.) that generated over $150 million in annual Medicare revenue while saving Medicaid $50 million per year. This has resulted in more patients being restored and going home. In that period of time, over forty thousand more patients had been discharged home than before. Not only does it improve the quality, it enables the nursing homes to fix the building and the parking lots, provide better working conditions to the staff, which improves morale, and lowers turnover and absenteeism. It truly is a win-win situation.

Jerry Rhoads's Paradigm Shift

In 1987 while running Fox Valley Rehabilitation Center, I was sent the classic court case that would change my career and life.

Fox v. Bowen **and** *Transmittal 262* **(Connecticut 1986); then** *Jimmo v. Sebelius* **was issued October 26, 2012 (Vermont 2012). Federal judges issued opinions that found the federal government in** violation of Title XVIII of the Social Security Act depriving the elderly, disabled, and infirm of their rightful Medicare benefits.

Where does the federal government stand on what we are doing? Is it gaming the system or committing fraud and abuse of the Medicare program? I was notified by Aetna Insurance Company that a court case had been issued in 1986 that would enable me to hold the Social Security Administration and the Department of Health and Human Services accountable to the Medicare insurance policy and what constitutes the obligation of Medicaid as the last resort for payment for nursing homes.

The use of *Fox v. Bowen* and *Transmittal 262* as the basis for providing the skilled services and documenting the physician and nurse involvement in the daily care the government must pay by law. Most providers and consultants are not schooled in this, nor do they know how to plan the care, deliver the care, and defend the claims. As a result, typically, the nursing homes are afraid to send the bill and opt to bill private resources then Medicaid instead. Since Medicare is the only pay source that pays for truly restoring the patients, they end up on welfare for the rest of their lives. This way, the facility loses money, the family loses their loved one, the patient loses hope, and the state Medicaid programs end up with bills they should not be paying.

For example, our client in Arkansas had Blue Cross of Arkansas as the fiscal intermediary. As we helped their thirteen facilities stop billing Medicaid inappropriately and billing Medicare, justifiably Blue Cross stopped payment on over two hundred claims, amounting to over $2 million. This was done in violation of *Fox v. Bowen* and *Transmittal 262*. An attorney for the provider brought this to Blue Cross's attorney, who advised the intermediary to pay the claims. Prior to that, we had appealed thirty-seven cases to the administrative law judges and won all of them. So in effect, the government was illegally withholding funds from the providers. We were not afraid to confront them and eventually prevailed. Over the last twenty years, my firm has done this a number of times where majority of the providers acquiesce and do not establish a claim. If and when the problem gets fixed nationally, most of the providers will be left out in the cold with Medicaid on their heels.

Why hasn't this problem been fixed? It will eventually when the masses realize that we have to restore the elderly, not just warehouse them in nursing homes. As predicted by this statement, the Center of Medicare Advocacy sued CMS for misapplying the Medicare entitlement to Part A coverage by challenging the use of improvement standard as a rule of thumb used for the purpose of denying entitled coverage to Medicare beneficiaries, bringing an end to Medicare's long-practiced but illegal application of an "improvement standard." The settlement of the case [*Jimmo v. Sebelius*, No. 5:11-cv-00017 (D. Vt.)] will improve access for tens of thousands of Americans, especially older adults and people with disabilities, whose Medicare coverage is denied or terminated because these beneficiaries are considered "not improving" or "stable." Resolution of this legal challenge effectively ends this harmful practice and ensures fair coverage rules for those who live with chronic conditions and rely on Medicare to cover basic, necessary health care.

Medicare should cover essential care for the treatment and management of chronic conditions. This settlement offers a real opportunity to finally eliminate the use of the unfair improvement standard to deny these claims.

Lead plaintiff Glenda Jimmo is a seventy-six-year-old resident of Bristol, Vermont. Blind since the age of nineteen, she is confined to a wheelchair as a result of her disabling conditions, including a below-the-knee amputation. She requires regular skilled-nursing services in her home to provide wound care and help manage her condition. She is proud to have had the opportunity to challenge this illegal Medicare policy and relieved to know that her care and the care for thousands of other older people and people with serious disabilities will be covered by Medicare.

"Filing the settlement agreement begins a long process to reverse the damage done to tens of thousands of Medicare beneficiaries with chronic conditions," observed plaintiffs' lead counsel, Gill Deford.

The court's tentative approval of the settlement will be followed by notification to the class members, who will have an opportunity to comment in writing and at a hearing on the proposed settlement, after which the judge will make her final decision on the settlement.

Under the proposed settlement, a nationwide class of beneficiaries will be certified, numerous parts of the *Medicare Benefit Policy Manual* will be rewritten, and CMS will carry out an educational campaign for providers, Medicare contractors, and adjudicators. The revised CMS manual language will clarify that Medicare coverage is available for maintenance services when skilled personnel are required to perform or supervise the care or therapy safely and effectively. In addition, many class members will have an opportunity to have their previously denied claims reviewed under the revised Medicare standards. Plaintiffs' attorneys will monitor and, if necessary, enforce the provisions of the agreement.

While the Centers for Medicare & Medicaid Services (CMS), which is the federal agency responsible for the Medicare program, continues to deny the existence of the rule of thumb known as the improvement standard, beneficiaries and advocates know that contractors and other adjudicators repeatedly rely on it to deny Medicare claims. Nationwide, thousands of cases of the illegal and unjust practice were identified in 2011 alone.

The lawsuit was brought in United States District Court in Burlington, Vermont, by seven individual plaintiffs from Vermont, Connecticut, Rhode Island, Maine, and Pennsylvania and seven national organizational plaintiffs: the National Committee to Preserve Social Security and Medicare, the National Multiple Sclerosis Society, Parkinson's Action Network, Paralyzed Veterans of America, the American Academy of Physical Medicine and Rehabilitation, the United Cerebral Palsy Association, and the Alzheimer's Association. The plaintiffs joined with the named defendant, secretary of health and human services Kathleen Sebelius, in asking the federal judge to approve the settlement of the case on October 16, 2012.

CHAPTER TWELVE

"GOTCHA" REGULATIONS MONOPSONY WINS AGAIN

ALL-AMERICAN RESTORATIVE CARE OF WASHINGTON

(Filed for Chapter 11 Bankruptcy Protection on December 19, 2013 Due to the State of Iowa's Action)

My wife, son, and I have been consultants in the retirement, nursing, and restorative home-care business for a combined one hundred years. When my wife Shari's mother passed away in a large corporate-owned nursing facility, Shari, my son, Kip, and I decided we can do better. We purchased two very run-down facilities, one here in Washington and one in Muscatine, Iowa. These two facilities were ready to close their doors; we cleaned them up, remodeled, and gave the facilities a physical face-lift, but more importantly than fresh paint, we implemented a fresh way of doing business.

During our two years and one month of ownership, we have lost $1 million in operating losses funded by bank debt, been fined $100,000, been defamed on the Internet by the State, smeared by the media for being a "special focus" dirtbag operator, while putting up with thirty days of surveyors on sight making things look worse than they are and arbitrarily enforcing capricious interpretations of the rules and preventing us from focusing on patient care, getting a fair hearing, and having due process of law. Why? Because our Muscatine facility and Washington were intended to be models of restorative care that would manage the elderly and disabled quality of life so they can return home, not their death in an institution. This would require the State change its Department of Inspections and Appeals (DIA) punitive enforcement strategy and stop bullying the small independent providers and scaring everyone in nursing homes with their gestapo tactics, civil money penalties, retaliation under their IDR Kangaroo Court, and CMS civil remedies using discounted fines to avoid appeals. Unless they are chains given a pass on the "good guy" list.

The two All-American Care facilities put the "homelike" in nursing home. In fact we don't even use the words *nursing home*; we use the words *restorative care* so we can discharge many back to their real home. We took over Muscatine four and one half years ago. Since then, they have sent 225 residents *back home* through restorative care. We have reduced the medication taken by residents by a combined 1/3. Sending patients back home and reducing their medication is unheard of in the nursing-home business, primarily because returning a patient out the door is sending income out the door. We didn't care; we conducted business to restore residents, giving them their life back. That was more important than keeping that person medicated.

In October 2011, we purchased the Washington facility to expand our restorative model to another location to further prove the premise. WASHINGTON CARE CENTER, LET'S LOOK BACK. (How would you like to have those prior owners back? How did they stay open for ten years? Did DIA make these improvements or try to destroy the mission of the new owners because of their views?)

1. 162 florescent bulbs burned out and not replaced—noncompliant
2. Eighty-six ballasts not replaced—noncompliant
3. Three halls of carpeting: filthy, never cleaned, bad odors—noncompliant
4. Total facility stunk and was dirty everywhere with junk in every room—noncompliant
5. Entire guest parking lot floods with each storm; sewer backed up without proper drainage—noncompliant
6. Brick building exterior built in late 1970s needed cleaned and painted—noncompliant
7. Old garage falling down with junk to the ceiling—noncompliant
8. Five dead trees in front—noncompliant
9. Entirely bad, leaking roof—noncompliant

10. Twenty-six security cameras installed to improve quality of care—exposed noncompliant activity
11. Old wooden signage falling down—noncompliant
12. All fifty windows had no blinds, and fifty-five rooms had old privacy curtains and ugly curtains that did not match—noncompliant
13. 125 beds in interior were dark, dank with urine odors—noncompliant
14. Three meals per day of bad food and cheap menus—noncompliant
15. Fourteen beds of a locked unit full of psych patients—noncompliant
16. Eighty employees for forty-eight patients was overstaffed with too many nurses, not enough CNAs with $100,000 in overtime—noncompliant
17. Inept administration—noncompliant
18. Locally a bad reputation, poor morale, and bad attitudes all acceptable to DIA—noncompliant

I offered to the governor in July 2011 and his director of Inspections and Appeals in August 2011 positive alternatives to their punitive and enforcement approach. In my opinion, that resulted in two years of retaliation for my views at our Washington facility.

DIA wants compliance from those that cannot fight back and let the larger chain operators get away with murder as did Washington Care Center and Muscatine Care Center before we took them over. After much success in Muscatine in implementing the restorative approach, the governor of Iowa visited and toured our facility in July 2011 with my emphasis on how this would save the State Medicaid program billions if Medicare would pick up their true share of the care. I then met with the director of DIA proposing the same approach, giving him and the governor white papers on the success that these methods had produced in Illinois. Then we purchased Washington in October 2011, and the retaliation began and has not stopped until they put us out of business. DIA put a hold on our admission four times during an eighteen-month period, forcing our census down from sixty to forty and costing us at least $1.4 million in annualized revenue.

The Rhoads family is on the verge of bankruptcy and has not been able to get an attorney that will help us fight the loss of our business, contrived by politicians and bureaucrats that say "Just comply" (and they let the prior owner of both Muscatine and Washington to operate despite numerous violations that far exceed what we have been alleged of), and hung before we have had our appeals adjudicated or heard by an unbiased court.

There are precedent setting cases that support our position. *Beechwood v. State of New York* who found the State guilty of retaliation against a skilled-nursing home operator and lost a settlement of $25 million; *Fox v. Bowen* and *Jimmo v. Sibelius* that found the federal government guilty of depriving the elderly of their Medicare benefits, but all attorneys are not willing to sue their friends at the State and would rather the small businesses go out of business regardless of the due process of law. This leads to the need for a provider bill of rights to make sure we follow due process of law.

***Last summer, a local Muscatine magazine wrote a story about our facility. The author wrote a very personal story about the difference between the care his grandfather received at the facility, years and years ago, under the old ownership—compared to the care his one hundred year-old grandmother currently receives under our ownership. The author claims it is night and day. Under the former ownership, you would walk in, and the smell would be unbearable. You would see residents sitting in the same spot, staring at the floor for hours. That wasn't a home. Sure, you got your pills on time, and your diaper changed. But that was it—pills and diapers, according to the government regulations. Fast-forward to how we run our facilities. The smell is long gone. All-American Care has a gym for physical therapy, movies, bingo, music, karaoke, discussion groups, and a garden area to enjoy being outside. Residents have a life here.

Everything sounds great, right? Patients are happy, enjoying their golden years, so what's the problem? Nursing homes have government oversight. The nursing-home industry hasn't seen innovation in twenty-five years. These regulations ensure the diapers are changed and the medication is distributed and meals are fed on time. But innovation in this business—the regulators aren't used to this kind of activity, and this has brought attention to All-American Care from the State of Iowa. It has brought fines and sanctions, even though countless families, like the author of that magazine article, are more than happy with the care of their family members, and most importantly, the patients are happier.

As an extension of the State of Iowa retaliation, the Washington, Iowa, facility recently had a resident pass away. The State of Iowa is fining All-American Care $78,000 for failure to attempt to resuscitate a patient, *after* the patient was dead. The Washington County medical examiner investigated the case, and they claimed the patient was in rigor mortis, body cyanotic, had passed body fluids, and therefore, CPR and the initiation of a code was *not* warranted. The family of the resident who passed away sent a letter telling us they were happy and satisfied with the care of their family member. Why then is the State fining us for not calling a code and performing CPR? The Washington County examiner and, most importantly, the family themselves don't have a problem, but somehow a bureaucrat in Des Moines has a problem with us? That doesn't make any sense.

This is the living proof of the bureaucrats destroying Americans' quality of life in nursing homes across the county, not protecting it. Nursing homes are not encouraged to be creative, innovative, and provide an actual home for people; they are motivated to simply play by the bureaucrat's rules, keep patients overly medicated, and collect their checks. We are concerned about quality of life! We will continue to be concerned about quality of life for our residents regardless of the bureaucrat sanctions.

Lauded Nursing Home Drew Citations 7 Weeks Earlier
Clark Kauffman, ckauffman@dmreg.com 12:18 a.m. CDT July 28, 2014

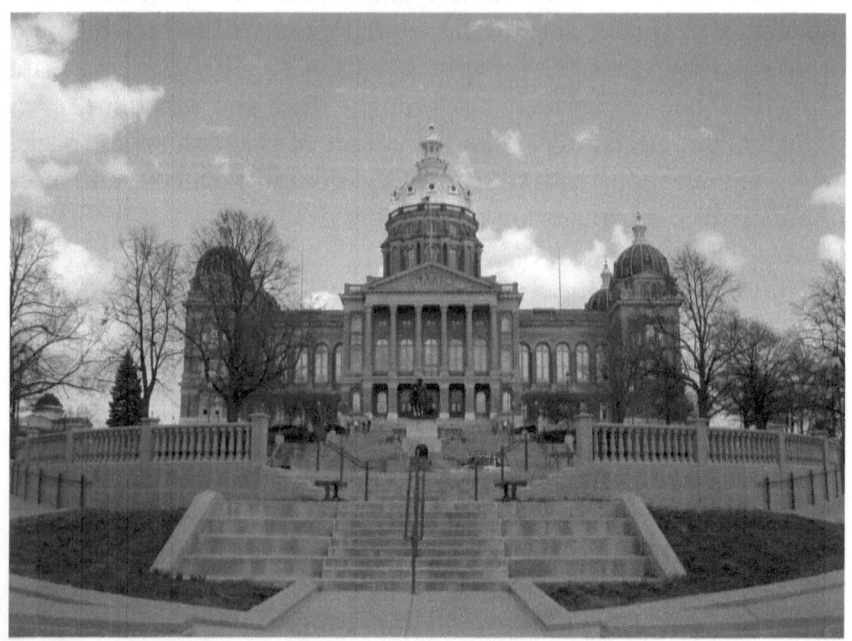

An eastern Iowa nursing home recognized by Gov. Terry Branstad as one of the best in the state was cited by inspectors seven weeks earlier for widespread unsanitary conditions and failure to meet residents' nutritional needs.

The 126-bed Woodland Terrace care facility in Waverly was written up May 13 for a variety of problems, including a food-preparation area that inspectors described as "highly soiled" and littered with dust, debris and discarded food.

Branstad's office announced July 9 that Woodland Terrace was one of three Iowa care facilities to receive the 2014 Governor's Award for Quality Care in Health Care Facilities. Christine Frederick of Clearwater, Fla., nominated the home for the honor, noting that her mother is a longtime resident of the facility and has received the best "physical, emotional and spiritual care."

"The fact that the nominator's loved one has resided in the Waverly facility for more than 13 years speaks volumes about the care provided by the Woodland Terrace staff," Lt. Gov. Kim Reynolds said in a news release announcing the award. "While conducting an on-site evaluation of the facility's nomination, staff from the Iowa Department of Inspections and Appeals were approached by numerous residents who praised the dedicated personnel and caring environment at the nursing home."

Branstad and Reynolds have repeatedly said that under previous administrations, Iowa's state regulators—and nursing home inspectors, in particular—embraced "a 'gotcha' attitude" that focused on punishing corporate violators instead of helping them improve and meet minimum standards. Branstad has credited his administration with changing that approach to regulation.

Dean Lerner, who headed the state inspections department under former Gov. Chet Culver, said the award is indicative of the Branstad administration's industry-friendly approach to regulation.

"The nursing home industry continues to be a significant, loyal contributor to Gov. Branstad's political campaigns," Lerner said. "If fines were imposed for these shameful conditions—and in an amount greater than the nursing homes' cost savings that created them—maybe residents wouldn't have to suffer."

According to state records, an inspection of Woodland Terrace's kitchen in early May revealed "highly soiled floors" littered with dust, food particles, paint chips, cookies, jelly and other debris. One area of the kitchen floor had three inches of an unidentified "dried substance," and kitchen carts were described as highly soiled with debris and food.

Inspectors said the food preparation counter was visibly soiled; window screens were highly soiled; a steam table was crusted with food and debris; plastic tubs used to store newly washed utensils contained a large amount of debris; ready-to-use appliances were soiled with dried pancake batter from meals served four days earlier; and a walk-in cooler was littered with shredded cheese, onion peels and debris.

Kitchen workers told inspectors they had no cleaning duties and no time to clean the area. The home's "executive chef," who was also in charge of maintaining a clean kitchen, told inspectors he ranked the quality of his work as a "3" on a scale of 1 to 10, with 10 being the best.

Inspectors reviewed five residents' diets and determined none had received the food they were supposed to be served according to their care plans. At one meal, for example, some residents received too little meat and protein, and some received none of the noodles and vegetables on the menu. Inspectors also determined that prior to being served, the food was not being kept at the recommended minimum temperature, with ground meat served at only 118 degrees.

No fines were imposed as a result of the inspectors' findings. Woodland Terrace has submitted a plan of correction outlining the steps taken to address the problems. The facility's CEO told inspectors the executive chef has left the home's employment and the other staff have been re-educated on food service.

A spokesman for Branstad declined to comment on the inspectors' findings until he could look into the matter further.

The Governor's Award for Quality Care is based on special programs and activities offered by the facilities, as well as each home's compliance with federal health care regulations.

Woodland Terrace was recognized in part for a pet therapy program that allows residents to socialize with Lucy, a specially trained black Labrador retriever.

In 2013, state inspectors cited Woodland Terrace for the legal agreement residents had to sign upon admission to the facility. That agreement made any individual who signed it—including third parties, such as family members—personally liable for cost of the resident's care.

At the time, inspectors also cited the home for inadequate infection control, saying that as they watched, the facility staff repeatedly failed to sanitize the glucose meter used to test residents' blood-sugar levels.

The other winners of the 2014 Governor's Award for Quality Care in Health Care Facilities were Friendship Haven in Fort Dodge and Prairie View Home in Sanborn.

Prairie View Home was last inspected in November. Inspectors reported no violations at the facility.

Friendship Haven was last inspected in November and was cited for failure to provide adequate incontinence care for residents; failure to adequately treat bedsores; and failure to keep food at the proper temperature before serving.

COULD IT BE THAT THE REGULATORS ARE SUBJECTIVE, ARBITRARY, CAPRICIOUS, AND BY ALL MEANS, CORRUPTED BY POLITICS AND THEIR CAMPAIGN FOR POWER?

CHAPTER THIRTEEN
ALL-AMERICAN RESTORATIVE CARE
Rhoads Family Personal History

Jerry Rhoads started his CPA business in Morton, Illinois, in 1977 specializing in nursing homes. He started development of software for clinical and financial applications in 1979 after raising venture capital to create his invention of Caregiver Management Information Systems. In 1984, he was forced to put the software in chapter 11 protection and moved his consulting business back to Chicago. Over the next twenty-five years he, his wife, and his son serviced nursing homes in many different ways and continued development of his dream clinical quality control–and-cost system.

In 1987, Jerry took over management of a 207-bed skilled-nursing center, Fox Valley Convalescent Center in Elgin Illinois. Troubled and decertified, he, as the administrator, turned the facility into a five-star quality program in thirteen months, and it was sold. He then took a contract from the Seventh Day Adventist group and did the same thing for Carington Convalescent Center a 206-bed facility in Glendale Heights, Illinois. During this period, Jerry developed an organizational structure that enabled him to improve the quality to a six-star rating by the State survey agency. He has published four books on this approach to managing outcomes for income, not the proverbial opposite.

After twenty years of implementing the Medicare management module of the Caregiver System, Jerry, his wife, Shari, and son, Kip, purchased a troubled and underperforming one-hundred-bed skilled facility in Muscatine, Iowa. This allowed Shari and Jerry to return to their home state and hopefully implement the whole system, not just the Medicare module. As the modernization and reconstitution of the facility took place over a four-year period, it became evident that the use of the Medicare module would, in fact, save the government millions of dollars due to its structured programming so patients could be returned home. In fact, it works so well that All-American Care of Muscatine has discharged 225 back into the community while sustaining an average census of over 85 percent—unheard of in today's competitive environment.

Jerry, having proven that his organizational structure and software could reduce overall cost of care and send more restored patients back home, invited the governor of Iowa to visit, which he did in July of 2011; he toured and got copies of Jerry's book and written materials. Jerry then met with the director of Inspections and Appeals for the State of Iowa to present the concept (documented in white papers) that the State go to a collaborative survey system to reinforce and help the providers to meet the quality standards proposed by the regulators and then pay for it with a "pay for performance" system to reward quality to replace the enforcement approach being used.

Jerry, Shari, and Kip, in the meantime, decided to build another outcome-based model in Washington, Iowa, acquired another troubled and likely-to-close facility of 125 beds with ninety licensed for skilled nursing in October of 2011—that is, when the damage hit the fan. A complaint survey by the very department that Jerry was trying to get to approach regulatory compliance in a more productive way converged on his facility in Washington.

Two very tumultuous years later, our very punitive, arbitrary, and capricious Department of Inspections and Appeals are maneuvering to close us down. How can they possibly contend that the enforcement tactics they have used on us improve anything but their arrogant attitude, that force will produce positive results? It hurts the staff, the patients, the families, the owners, and the taxpayers who are funding this gestapo tactic and tearing down the fabric of the small independent operators who do not have the political clout that the large chains in the state do through the Iowa Health Care Association and their lobbyists.

The Biggest Bully

We acquired the Washington facility October 10, 2011, from a Des Moines–based operator that had written if off and had allowed it to sink into a flooded parking lot with 160 fluorescent bulbs burnt out and eighty-seven ballasts that did not function, leaving the facility dark, dank, and smelly. As we had already done in Muscatine, we painted an ugly red brick building white, named it the DC Whitehouse, after Shari Rhoads's mother Dorotha C. White, who was prematurely abused and killed in a nursing home in Lake Zurich, Illinois. In her memory, we had decided on the white building and business that would restore the elderly and disabled, not just warehouse them, as is typically done in the long-term care business.

The facility literally was sitting on five acres that was fronted by dead trees, had odors permeating the building, rooms filled with junked beds, wheelchairs, commodes, mattresses, and walkers that were unsanitary and never to be used again. It took over a year to clean up the inside, clean out the junk. It took seventeen truckloads to the junk dealers to get the facility in any kind of operating shape that, need I remind you, the surveyors had let function in that manner for ten years. The previous administration had been told by the surveyors on one occasion to tear down all the window blinds while they went to lunch to punish them for a patient hanging themselves to death with a blind cord; no fines nor threatened civil penalties. The facility was mistreating patients and families with no enforcement being done because the owner had ten other facilities and had an in with the State.

There were violations everywhere, and we were in the process of fixing the interior as well as the exterior, evaluating staff and getting to know the families when in late December 2011 (two months after we took over this very noncompliant disaster), our friendly surveyor showed up with a complaint about the heat and staff sleeping in the Alzheimer's unit. However, on complaints, the surveyors are allowed to look for other violations, and Mr. Rob Reck certainly took advantage of that authority.

He looked into falls and found out from interviews with the staff that there had been one in the unit. Six weeks later, thousands of pages of copies and a surveyor on a seek-and-destroy "*gotcha*" mission, we received sixty-some pages of allegations, $20,000 in fines and were put into a special-focus category that designated us for closure unless we were reblessed with three clean surveys and avoided all complaints until they came back out to do the revisit on the enforcement rules that allowed them to publish all the violations on the Internet before we had exercised our rights to appeal the Des Moines *Register*'s Clark Kauffman, self-designated nursing-home hater then smeared us all over the state with his slander and defamation of the facts.

The fall in the unit was caught on our video security system that we installed to protect the patients, staff, and ourselves from being accused of the very thing Mr. Reck was accusing us of substandard care and not properly supervising our staff (two months after we took over a facility that they let violate every standard there was for ten years). We went through all the appeal hoops, waited for one and half years for an opinion from an administrative law judge who slept through much of the hearing, allowing the federal and state government attorneys to tamper with the videos by combining five clips into one showing that our staff did nothing for forty-eight minutes to respond to the fallen patient when, in fact, the patient was a behavior problem, used to lying on the floor as a coping mechanism, and had the staff standing down until she had more than one CNA or nurse to approach her. Rob Reck, the surveyor, continually perjured himself with unsupported testimony on the condition of the patient and the accuracy of the videos. The ensuing punitive action rejected the staff testimony as not being documented in writing. Our fines of $20,300 were enforced, we stayed in special focus and experienced four different holds on admissions and two conditional licenses that allowed the surveyors full rein over our facility.

Then in September, Jerry Rhoads, frustrated by the punitive actions taken against him and his businesses, announced he planned to run for governor to deal with this situation and the impact of Obama Care for which he has expertise. The following week, the surveyors were in to answer a complaint by a former employee who we believe was stealing from us and went straight for an expired patient, alleging we should have performed CPR even though he had been dead for up to thirty minutes. In the chart, the patient, two years earlier, signed to be a full code, and the staff knew of that status but did not perform it due to his obvious rigorous condition. Without regard to the attending physician, medical examiner, family, and the medical director stating it was inappropriate, the inspectors concluded, with much evidence to the contrary, that the patient was still alive and was abused by staff for not performing CPR. The facility was given an immediate jeopardy violation, fined $78,000, and put on admissions hold for the fourth time in a year with DIA and CMS threatening closure if administration did not present what they termed missing policies and procedures for such a situation even though such were in place and the staff ignored them.

We were warned by our counsel that the State would retaliate if we appealed their allegations, which certainly turned out to be true.

CHAPTER FOURTEEN

BIGGEST BULLY TRICK: THE DEATH OF ENTERPRISE

The allegation related to Dependent Adult Abuse is theorizing that Richard T. was still alive when the nurses decided not to perform CPR and they caused his death. There is no proof that Mr. Richard T's clinical death was reversible.

Reversal of Clinical Death: Per Dr. Robin Plattenberger, Medical Examiner "regarding death of Richard T., on 6/2/2013. According to my investigation the deceased was in rigor mortis, body cyanotic and had passed body fluids. The initiation of code not warranted".

STAGES OF DEATH AND RIGOR MORTIS

1. **(On June 1, 2013, Richard had just returned from the hospital, near death, with sepsis, and Michael Carl, LPN, sent him back to the hospital with a 103 temperature, to be admitted, but the hospital sent him back and would not readmit him. He died the next morning, June 2, between 6:00 a.m. and 6:20 a.m.; there was no evidence of cardiac arrest or distress. Per the death certificate, the estimated time of death reported by Teresa Burley was 6:35 a.m. of arterial sclerosis).** "Between 6:00 and 6:20 a.m., Richard's heart stops and his brain starts to die within 4 to 6 minutes at 6:00 to 6:10 a.m. and again at 6:20 a.m. Michelle, LPN, charge nurse and Teresa, LPN were asked by Heidi a nurse assistant to go look at his breathing" (*Medical Journals*, AHA).
2. No vital signs and breathing stops. At 6:30 a.m. Teresa, LPN, checked for vital signs. Teresa listened to his lungs, heart, redial pulse, "There was nothing." Jacob, CNA, who went to the room with Heidi said, "His color was pale and he was

not breathing." Jacob felt he had been dead for one hour / was yellowish-white in color.
3. Skin turns gray. Michelle, LPN, said his color was blue-green and he was having trouble breathing at 5:30 a.m.
4. Muscles relax. At 6:30 a.m. Jacob and Heidi, CNAs, found him nonresponsive.
5. Bladder and bowels will empty. Virginia, LPN noticed that the patient's face was ashen in color and was passing fluids. Michelle G., CNA, body fluids were on the bed, Michelle, LPN, did everything, turned Richard and BM, urine were expelled.
6. Body temp will drop. Michelle G., CNA, said he was discolored, clammy, and not breathing.
7. After thirty minutes, skin gets purple and waxy. Michelle G., CNA, "He was bluish in color, clammy."
8. Lips, finger- and toenails fade to pale. Teresa, LPN, "His color was ashen whitish/yellow."
9. Blood pools at lower part of body leaving bruises. Jacob, CNA, "He was molting." Michelle G., CNA, said, "Richard had passed all bodily fluids" when she entered the room around 6:30 a.m.
10. Hands and feet turn a bluish color. Michelle, RN, said, "His color was blue-green."
11. Muscles start to tighten. Michelle G., CNA, said, "Richard was stiff in upper area and shoulders."
12. Eyes start to sink in the skull. Jacob states he is nonresponsive at 6:30 a.m.
13. Rigor mortis is setting in, in a matter of thirty minutes. At 6:35 a.m. Michelle, LPN, asked Teresa, LPN, if he was gone, and Teresa said yes. Teresa said she did not think about looking for code since Michelle told her he had come back here to die.
14. Richard T. died between the hours of 6:00 and 6:20 a.m., June 2, 2013.
15. At 6:30 a.m., according to the American Heart Association, medical examiner, attending physician, medical director, and CMS standards of quality directive, CPR would be contra indicated.

Per Dick T. Sr., Richard T's father, "Richard did not want to have CPR, and we don't believe it was necessary because of his condition when found by the nurses."

All three nurses on duty had access to the patient charts that were plainly marked with a 1 by 4 inch label on the spine since March 2013: *red* (stop) DNR or *green* (go full code) CPR that constitutes a system of procedures for the nurses. Our policy since we acquired the facility is that there is a code-status sheet just inside (front) of the chart and was in place for this patient each time he was readmitted. Your survey staff had access to the charts and should have verified our system, policies, and procedures as being in compliance without arbitrary allegations put in the 2567. In our investigation, the nurses decided that the patient was in rigor mortis and did feel it was inappropriate to perform CPR.

Michelle Alexander, LPN, charge nurse, has worked here for seven years and did know Richard's code status, and she knew where to look for it in his chart. Basic knowledge for nurses is to look in the chart for the code status. Michelle was asked by Heidi, a nurse assistant, to go look at his breathing, and she said she had just looked at him fifteen minutes ago and he had no problem breathing at 5:30 am and she was ready to clock out.

Nursing judgment would tell you that anyone could have a change in condition any minute. She did not get up to go to check. Heidi, CNA, repeated her request. Teresa gathered the equipment, and she and Michelle went down to the patient's room at 6:30 a.m. They checked for vital signs, and there were none. He was in the early stages of rigor mortis, and Michelle said his color was blue-green. She asked Teresa if he was gone, and Teresa said yes. Michelle went to comfort the aide standing in the hall crying. Then Michelle came back to the door of the room and asked Teresa if she wanted her to call the family, and Dr. Teresa said yes.

Teresa Burely, LPN, came to work, per the time clock, at 6:20 a.m., was at the nurses' station for report from Michelle A., when Heidi, a nurse assistant, came and said the patient "was not breathing right."

Michelle said he was having no problem breathing at 5:30 a.m. Then Heidi repeated the request to have a nurse come to the room and examine him since he did not seem to be breathing. Michelle and Teresa went to his room. Teresa listened to his lungs, heart, radial pulse; there was nothing, and his color was ashen whitish/yellow, and he was passing fluids, a sign of rigor mortis. Michelle asked if he was gone, and Teresa said yes. Michelle left the room to console the aide in the hallway. Teresa said, when Michelle didn't come back, she decided that she didn't need to perform CPR. When Michelle came back, she told her to go pass her medications, and she (Michelle) was calling family and attending physician.

(At 7:00 a.m., Susie Davis, director of nursing, was called and queried Michelle A. if they had performed CPR and called the medical examiner, and she stated they had called the family and it was not necessary.)

Virginia Miller, LPN, came to work at 6:00 a.m., received report from Michelle, prepared her cart, and went to hall 6 to begin doing her blood sugar checks. At 7:00 a.m., Virginia was told by Heidi the patient had passed away. She then went to the patient's room, and there were two aides already in the process of preparing the body for viewing by the family. She noticed that the patient's face was ashen in color and the body was passing fluids.

Jacob and Heidi (aides) went to Richard's room to get him up at 6:30 a.m. and found him nonresponsive, his color was pale, and he was not breathing. Jacob rubbed his chest and put his hand beneath his nose to see if he was breathing, and he was not, while Heidi went crying out of the room to get a nurse.

Michelle Gierloff, an aide, went to Richard's room, said he was discolored, clammy, and not breathing, came out and asked the nurse, "What do we do?" was told to go to hall 3, then fifteen minutes later, was asked to go clean Richard up. The body fluids were on the bed; Richard was stiff in the upper area and shoulders.

We have talked with the patient's family (father and brother), and they have stated that they wouldn't have wanted CPR done, and they know the patient wouldn't have wanted it, especially in his condition. The family's past experience with the patient's mother was that when CPR was done, she had broken ribs, was put on a respirator, and the balance of her life was horrible. They also said they were happy with the care and loved that we had always given Richard great care and that he also loved it here and loved us. We have enclosed our conversations with Richards' father. He asked Susie if she would just write it as he said it—he is eighty and said his writing was awful, so she did, and had him sign it. I (Sharon Rhoads, administrator) was witness to his narration and signing.

SUMMATION:

This allegation related to dependent-adult abuse is theorizing that he was still alive when the nurses decided not to perform CPR and they caused his death. The tag and surrounding resulting IJ with civil penalties totaling $48,000 allege patient abuse, even to the extent of requiring the abuser to be separated from the abused patient who is clearly dead—this position is not supported by the facts.

Also, we have since been ordered by a directive from DIA to report the nurses to the nursing board for punishment. There is no evidence to support this theory. Our investigation proves that he died between the hours of 6:00 a.m. and 6:10 a.m. of natural causes and was in the early stages of rigor mortis not requiring CPR or heroic procedures.

We have sent in the previous submission a copy of the death certificate and a copy of statements from the medical examiner and staff involved in the incident. We plan to bring witnesses to that affect. Our witnesses will include a nurse, a CNA, a physician, and the director of nursing, who will testify to the facts regarding this erroneous allegation.

Recent Press and Media Conference Release

For Immediate Release
3:00 p.m. CDT; November 20, 2013 TODAY

All-American Care of Washington
601 E. Polk Street, Washington, Iowa

Publicist for **All-American Care**

Federal and State Regulators Ready to Deal Death Blow to Family-Owned Care Facility

Because CPR was not performed by nurses on a dead man.

A small family owned restorative care facility in Washington, IA was informed via telephone by the **Iowa Department of Inspections and Appeals** in collaboration with **The Centers of Medicare & Medicaid** Services that they are being punished and could close as a result of their investigation into an alleged patient abuse by All-American Care staff. Regulators imposed a fine of $78,000 plus $250 per day until they are re-inspected; all prior to the facility exercising its appeal rights.

As proven in the past these appeal rights are capriciously adjudicated by the same regulators that impose these very severe allegations that the Department of Inspections and Appeals publishes on the Internet to be picked up by the media for public dissemination and defamation of the owners.

Shari, her husband Jerry and son Kip Rhoads own and operate restorative care facilities in Muscatine and Washington IA. They are a couple in their early 70s who decided to try and make a difference in the health care industry after they watched, helplessly, the death of Shari's mother at the hands of a large corporate owned nursing facility. So they purchased two run down, ready to close the doors facilities and proceeded to modernize and clean them up, restore patient care and try to run a business in an industry controlled by large corporations plagued by patient abuse and neglect.

The Rhoads', with over 100 years combined experience in the health care industry, are no strangers to what is the Judge, Jury and sometimes Hangman capabilities of the Federal and State regulators. The Washington facility, which has been targeted under a special focus designation since 2012, was just about to get taken off probation for a previous alleged incident concerning a psych patient and the facility's video security cameras, when this elderly man's untimely death occurred.

According to Mr. Rhoads, the Department of Inspections and Appeals is controlled by regulators who have no real oversight or accountability whatsoever. They are free to bully the staff as they want and whatever they decide, goes. This has to Stop. With this latest action we may be forced to close the doors here in Washington and terminate over 50 dedicated employees. The worst part is the patients here will have to be relocated to unfamiliar surroundings away from family and in several cases will result in a premature death, especially the Alzheimer's patients.

Mr. Rhoads says his other facility, which is in compliance with State and Federal regulations, has also been targeted since his announcement to run for Governor. Unlike so many facilities that merely warehouse their patients until they pass away, the Rhoads' facilities have, in the short time he has operated them, have actually been able to restore 250 patients and return them to their *real homes*.

CHAPTER FIFTEEN
PUNISHMENT FOR LOSING MONOPSONY GAME

Congress of the United States
House of Representatives

COMMITTEE ON OVERSIGHT AND GOVERNMENT REFORM

2157 RAYBURN HOUSE OFFICE BUILDING

WASHINGTON, DC 20515–6143

MAJORITY (202) 225-5074
FACSIMILE (202) 225-3974
MINORITY (202) 225-5051

http://oversight.house.gov

1. Why does the CMS rating system allow nursing homes of average quality, as determined by government health inspectors, to receive overall ratings of five stars?

2. What is the status of CMS efforts to implement the Affordable Care Act provision requiring the use of payroll data to verify the accuracy of nursing home staffing levels?

3. What is the status of CMS efforts to implement an audit program to verify the accuracy of nursing home quality measures?

4. What other metrics are being considered? Has CMS considered the use of a consumer protection hotline or website to receive complaints about nursing homes to better inform the rating system?

5. What are the most significant benefits and challenges with incorporating fines and other enforcement actions by state authorities, as well as complaints filed by consumers with state agencies?

6. What are current CMS plans for introducing similar five-star rating systems for hospitals, dialysis centers, and home-health-care agencies, including the data to be used, the sources of the data, how the data will be verified, and the frequency of the data collection?

7. What improvements in nursing home care have resulted from the implementation of the rating system? What efforts have been made to review the impact of the rating system on nursing home care quality, and what findings have been reported?

Sincerely,

Elijah E. Cummings
Elijah E. Cummings
Ranking Member

My name is Jerry L. Rhoads
Owner of All-American Care
Muscatine and Washington Iowa

My wife, son and I currently own two skilled nursing facilities in Muscatine and Washington, Iowa and purchased a facility in Little Rock. We purchased them after 20 years of consulting with 150 skilled nursing facilities around the country. Our services were focused on getting the elderly their Medicare benefits so they could return home and not malinger in nursing homes on Medicaid.

We thought we could make a difference at the grass roots of long term care. We named them after my wife's mother Dorotha C. White and call them the DC Whitehouse in her memory. She was killed by a nursing home in Lake Zurich Illinois while we were out helping other facilities deal with the regulatory night mare we now term CMS and the Iowa Department of Inspections and Appeals the "Gotcha system" that emulates enforcement at its worst.

If you want to know what is wrong with the current 5 star rating system start asking the Administrators who are in fear of the surveyors and how arbitrarily and Capricious they are. They can and do ignore due process of law and the Administrative Procedures Act because Congress had made this into a negative ineffective weapon that they use very discriminatorily where the Government is immune from legal action and the providers are guilty until proven innocent.

After buying our first facility in Muscatine Iowa we began to get our Baptism in why the surveyors selectively get you if you question their authority. So I thought if we had more it would make a difference since I had been told that the small independent providers could not make it like the big chains due to political influence of campaign contributions and other corrupt cronyism.

We had great aspirations of showing the Governor of Iowa and his henchman Director of Inspections and Appeals how we could save Medicare and Medicaid billions by implementing restorative care in the skilled nursing facilities with the incentive being discharge to community based programs. We have proved this in Muscatine by discharging 57% back home. But oh no, that was not good enough, because we also suggested that they pay incentives for discharge not just assessment and treatment. Since the current reimbursement program that is being implemented for Medicaid across the country pays more for illness our rate goes down if we get the patients more functional and able to have a life outside of institutionalization.

Now we are selling the two facilities we put this in because of the enforcement system that the academics have imposed on the operators who really care for improving the quality of life not just how diapers are changed and pills are passed. I can guarantee you that every patient (resident) is being over medicated due to the waste of unnecessary and excessive medications costing the Medicare and Medicaid programs billions in costs and the functionality of patients that could return to the community but are not. Also after 40 years of enforcement we still have the same problems with accountability and poor results because the tactics are not collaborative or positive in intent. Our good regulators have been given the hammer and the use it discriminately and it is putting the mom and pops out of business and allowing the chains to dictate what your committee is bound and determined to do…nothing but more of the same…blame the small providers who cannot fight back

Let me, as an expert in this having spent all my career in trying to solve the dichotomy between services, cost and outcome, answer your

7 questions from the real world where the improvements have come from; the private sector:

1. CMS' five star counts mistakes and does not measure quality of life or outcomes. It was devised by PhD's who have never run any business let alone the hardest business there is ... a 24/7 skilled nursing facility anywhere in the country. It again has enforcement as its tactic not collaboration...it threatens income not pursuit of true outcomes.
2. Where does CMS get its all-important payroll data for enforcing some kind of staffing standards. Staffing is only a part of the pursuit of outcome. SNF's are paid on assessment (input) not on results (outcome) because the academics don't know an outcome from a hammer in the closet. In my book "Restore Elder Pride" enclosed with this letter is the definition of outcome and how output units of service are the way to motivate SNF's to provide restorative outcomes.
3. The CMS quality measures movement is negative counting of mistakes by the SNF's not measuring the functionality of patients and paying for output units of improvement and discharge. It pays for input assessment and more pills and wheelchairs.
4. More enforcement will never solve the problem and after 40 years of threats and fines we still have substandard care. We need to measure restorative processes not treatment and re-hospitalizations. Those are only symptoms of the real problem. The real problem is there are no real incentives to get the patients better and out...according to the operators there is nothing worse than an empty bed. In my facilities an empty bed is an outcome and more will come if they are assured you are going to restore them to their highest level of functioning and back to their families or to a higher quality of life if they have to remain in the nursing facility. It is a billion dollars cheaper to restore rather than implore.
5. I reiterate...the enforcement tactics don't work and never will. Try to run a business when the Government has all

the authority. I have proposed in my books and writings a Provider Bill of Rights when it comes to fines and complaints because the "Gotcha System" is designed to generate fines and honors all complaints equally even if it is from a terminated disgruntled employee that the surveyors call upon to dig up dirt on the SNF. How do I know this, well it put us out of business in our three facilities. Not only were the complaints blown out of proportion but concocted to punish me for fighting back.

6. The only system that has been developed that works is the Illinois six star system for skilled nursing facilities (I refer to this in my book). It was implemented with my help in the 1980's by the Department of Public Health and was called the QUIP program. It measures results not input units of mistakes and inaccurate metrics for quality of care and life. The six stars was an annual survey in six areas of outcome where the surveyors measured performance on those criteria that could be defined as contributing to the patients' welfare and functionality. The corresponding reimbursement system then paid for the add-on programs of restorative care that generated the six star results. It then paid an economic incentive for each star earned and paid retroactive bonuses based on that collaborative accountability system. Therefore, the six star facilities were truly the best in the state. I took over two no star facilities and turned them around by focusing the staff on attaining the six stars. Those providers who did not attain that status were incentivized to pursue each star and become the best. This system was thrown out by the Illinois Legislature because the big noncompliant owners did not want that accountability and distinction as a one or two star facility. This system works.

7. What improvements have resulted from the implementation of the CMS five star "Gotha System" ... my two facilities are one and two stars because the system punishes those that fight it. My staff, patients and families regard the system as a joke as it is. They think we are the best of the best (All-American Care) not slaves to CMS and DIA.

In summary, I have been in health care since 1962 through Kennedy, Johnson, Nixon, Carter, the Bushes, Clinton and now Obama either as a consultant to HEW on Medicare, the Associations on Medicaid or my clients and my patients trying to get CMS to comply with due process, and the regulations not interpretive guidelines . I am the most qualified person in the country to voice my opinion and I cannot get on any committees anymore because I am private sector and not a professor and/or PhD. But I am an advocate for enterprising Americans that can fix anything without punitive enforcement as the incentive.

I propose that your committee have me come before you with proof of what I propose and testify on your pertinent questions. My book should be required reading for your committee and all who proclaim to be experts on enforcement and civil money penalties as the way negative incentives get better results.

Very truly yours,
All-American Care
2002 Cedar Street Muscatine, Iowa
601 E. Polk Street Washington, Iowa

Jerry L. Rhoads, CPA, FACHCA
jrhoads@allamericancare.com
847/309-3946
1919 Wildwood Lane
Muscatine Iowa 52761

PS: Reprehensive Hayes I will call you if I do not hear from you or your staff.

From December 23, 2011, two months and twelve days after we took over a very noncompliant facility, we have had thirty-six visits or interventions by DIA; 4,999 copies of records and pages of interview with staff, former staff, families, and patients; three IDR hearings; one ALJ hearing; one meeting in Des Moines with DHS, CMS, and DIA; and a telephone call from CMS threatening closure. No patient was injured other than a bump on the head for the floor incident and one broken hip due to a fall; no significant wounds were found by the State's consultant, and

- $104,000 in fines,
- $70,000 in legal fees,
- $1.4 million lost revenue due to the two admission holds and two conditional license allowing no admissions,
- defamation of Kip Rhoads by publishing an allegation regarding sexual contact with a delusional patient without investigating the fabricated incident that put Kip in the hospital with high blood pressure,
- defamation of the Rhoads family by the Des Moines *Register* and local news media without due process of law,
- census rose to sixty from forty-seven with no Medicare program in place to sixty with twelve on Medicare by February survey hold that bottomed out at forty in mid-2012 and rose back up to fifty-four mid-2013 and is now back down to forty due to the nine months of admission holds imposed in the two years and three months we have owned the Washington facility, causing a loss of $1.4 million in revenue, creating $726,000 in operating losses in 2012, and $174,000 operating losses in 2013. Due to the $1 million financial borrowing that it took to keep the doors open, we have been forced to file chapter 11 bankruptcy for both the Washington operation and the Muscatine facility. The Rhoadses are being forced to sell both facilities as a result of the punitive actions by the State of Iowa Department of Inspections and Appeals (DIA) in retaliation for appeals and disagreements with the governor and the director of DIA.

All this in the mode of entrapment and punishment with no regard for due process. Nothing constructive has come from any of these actions.

In September, Jerry Rhoads announced his third-party bid for governor, citing the actions of state inspectors at All-American Restorative Care as one example of government interference.

> On his political website, Rhoads says it is his "mission to change the punitive and negative disincentives that exist in the federal and state [inspection] process to a reinforcement approach that allows the small businesses to direct their own version of quality of life."
>
> He says nursing homes are the "most regulated business of all time," and he calls for a shift in "spending away from enforcement to pay for collaborative rules and regulations."
>
> Gov. Terry Branstad has also said "Iowa should replace what he calls the gotcha attitude of state nursing-home inspectors with what he calls a more collaborative approach to regulation and oversight".
>
> Ha-ha — HE lied again. He continued to do the same punitive , gotcha system with the same gotcha surveyors with the same bad results ... it is not about the patients, it is all about enforcement at any cost to the providers. Monopsony operating at its worst.

CHAPTER SIXTEEN
HOW TO STOP THE BULLY

Beechwood Nursing Home Settlement Reached
by Seth Voorhees

The state of New York will have to pay the former owner of a Rochester nursing home $25 million. The payment is part of a federal court settlement, after jurors found state health officials improperly retaliated against the owner of the facility in shutting the place down more than a decade ago.

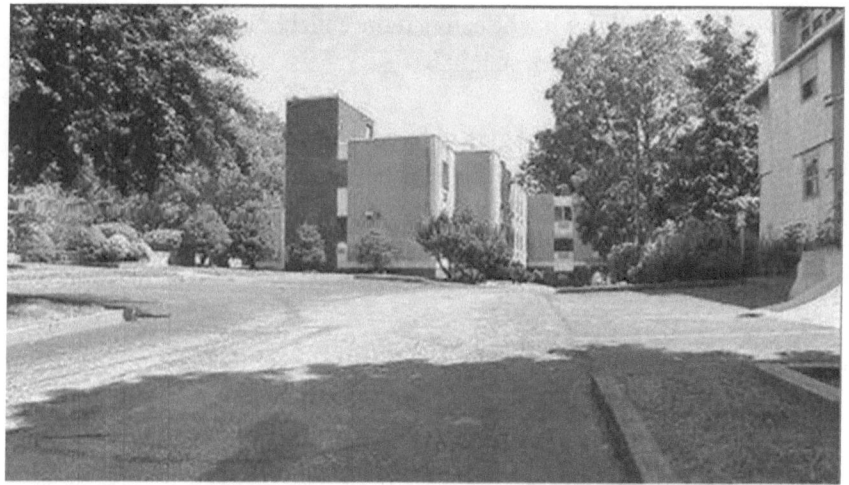

900 Culver Road is boarded up. Empty. Under lock and key.

Former owner Brook Chambery can hardly stand to drive by.

"I try not to. It's hard to look at."

Go back to 1999. That's when the New York State Department of Health shut down Beechwood Restorative Care Center and took Chambery's license to run it.

"I basically consider it a raid on the facility," he said.

The state accused Chambery of neglect and poor patient care. But Chambery fought back, saying some in the Department of Health had an axe to grind because he'd been an outspoken critic of state policy.

"It's not nice to get your name slandered out there or be accused of harming patients, or for my staff . . . they were just annihilated by this whole event."

On Wednesday, a federal judge announced a settlement under which the state must pay Chambery $25 million. A seven-week trial resulted in a jury siding with Chambery.

"It's nice that it's been ended. I get on with my life. My reputation is restored," Chambery said.

"Key people in the DOH wrote back to one another about Beechwood going down," said Kevin Cooman, Chambery's lawyer of 13 years. "'Amen' and 'hallelujah,' which was responded to by saying 'hot diggity dog!'"

Cooman says the case and its outcome holds the state accountable.

"This is a clear case where the Department of Health overstepped its bounds and authority for clearly vindictive personal reasons to attack a thriving, innovative business," Cooman said.

After the state shut down his nursing home, Chambery took up what he calls another full-time job, albeit not one with immediate payoff: fighting to win the case, and clear his name.

"To realize why I've been doing this these 13 years you'd have to have lived through those three months back in 1999," Chambery said.

The state had requested the Chambery's receive just one dollar. A lawyer for the State Attorney General's Office referred us to a spokesperson in Albany, who didn't respond to a request for comment.

"So it's been a long hard road," Chambery said.

Chambery's parents opened Beechwood in 1955. He basically grew up there. He says the settlement vindicates not only his family, but his former staff, but it won't bring back what's been lost.

"It was a horrid thing. A horrid thing to live through."

CHAPTER SEVENTEEN
BIGGEST BULLY IN IOWA

THE GOVERNOR

January 21, 2011 (updated to January 25, 2012)

Honorable Terry Branstad, Governor
Office of the Governor, State Capitol
1007 East Grand Ave.
Des Moines, IA 50311

Dear Governor Branstad:

My wife and I are originally from Indianola, Iowa and I am a graduate of Simpson College, class of '61. After graduation I was recruited by Arthur Andersen & Co. and moved to Chicago. I am a CPA and a licensed Nursing Home Administrator in Iowa, Illinois, Arkansas.

My purpose in writing you is to elicit help in our mission to improve the quality of service to the elderly in nursing homes. I personally have been involved in health care since 1962 as a consultant, an accountant and now operator. My wife, son and I own All-American Care of Muscatine a skilled nursing facility in Muscatine Iowa. We bought it 16 months ago and have restored it externally and internally using what we call the Restorative Model of care. We now have a similar project in Washington, Iowa.

We utilize computer technology to assess the patients being admitted far beyond the limited Minimum Data Set (MDS 3.0) that the State of Iowa requires. Our experience collectively transcends 5 decades, 22 states and 140 nursing facilities with our consulting and software technology. We designed it and programmed the processes so the clinical services could be standardized so we could assign the work to the staff, cost the care and measure performance based on problem resolution not averages produced by the MDS.

Since taking over the Muscatine facility we have admitted 24 patients in 2009, 94 patients in 2010, (390 admitted through December 31, 2013 with 241 discharged back home) this is unheard of in the typical nursing home therefore, we are not the typical nursing home. We have designed and implemented the Restorative Model to replace the ineffective "Medical Models" and "Social Models" that continue to frustrate regulators and families.

We have done this on our own volition since CMS only engages academic institutions in their demonstration projects to prove what they have already decided. Everything must be budget neutral and administratively simple. Well neither outcome is ever attained and we dig the hole deeper when the solutions are enterprise models not political models.

What I propose is to link the ineffective survey process to reimbursement and reimbursement to outcome. Our software does that now and needs to be used in a demonstration mode. Please see the white paper attached for that project.

Thank you for visiting our facility in Muscatine so you could see for yourself the difference between what we are doing and what others are doing.

I also understand that you personally doubt the effectiveness of the current enforcement approach that CMS has for survey policies and procedures. We had an annual survey last year and had 3 F-Tags and 1 K-Tag and 7 pages of deficiencies this year after turning over 60 staff members to improve our services we get an annual survey with 14 K-tags and 11 F-tags with 60 pages of incrimination. It is totally punitive and is killing the goose. If we have improved the outcomes and this is not the result of the survey process then it is a waste of time and State taxpayer dollars.

28 pages of that deficiency report focused on how our staff inappropriately wipes patients bottoms when they dirty themselves

not one page on how our restorative teams are getting patients more functional so more can go home and our psycho/social programming is allowing depressed patients to become socially and emotionally involved in our clubs, classes and group therapy. The surveyors say we do not qualify for the best practices designation wow is that a joke. As is the CMS 5 star program that only counts mistakes not outcomes.

The prior operator of this facility had let it go so far downhill that we spent $350,000 in remodeling costs and another $200,000 in improving the equipment and staffing only to be shot down by surveyors that only look at their interpretation of frivolous treatment and not outcomes. They are not even looking at the discharges or the improved functionality of our patients just ask the facilities and visitors who say "thank God you are not one of those smelly, careless nursing homes."

In our opinion unless enforcement is not turned into re-enforcement more and more money will be wasted on making the situation worse than it is and it is now unsustainable.

Very truly yours,

THE RHOADS FAMILY

_____ Jerry L. Rhoads, CEO

_____ Sharon K. Rhoads, VP

_____ Kip A. Rhoads, VP

Attached: Pursuit of Outcomes (a 6 star survey)

GOVERNOR BRANSTAD'S RESPONSE: no comment due to impending appeals.

"The creatures outside looked from pig to man, and from man to pig, and from pig to man again: but already it was impossible to say which was which." George Orwell's classic book on the Russian Revolution has become an intimate part of contemporary culture. It is an account of the transformation of Manor Farm into Animal Farm, of the brave struggle on the part of the animals to create a wholly democratic society built on the credo that all animals are created equal. Of course, as with its many counterparts in modern society, this brave struggle results in socialism, then Communism, then a new totalitarian regime and a new maxim: **"But some animals are more equal than others."**

Are some Iowa nursing home operators more equal than others ... ask Governor Brandstad who ignored how his Department of Inspection and Appeals violated the Administrative Procedures Act and the Rule of Law to quiet the Rhoadses and their innovative nursing homes that would save the Medicaid budget and improve the quality of life of our elderly nationwide.

Terry Branstad is not unfamiliar with bully pulpit tactics ... after 4 going on 5 terms in the Governor's bully pulpit he knows how to throw his weight around ... if isn't having the highway patrolman fired for a ticket after directing his driver to speed it's the dozen post office buildings he admittedly owns that he says are not a conflict of interest ... he certainly is comfortable with using his power for money.

CHAPTER EIGHTEEN
HOW TO WIN THE MONOPSONY GAME AND DEFEAT THE BIGGEST BULLY

WHY ARE WE LOSING THE MONOPSONY GAME

READ MY LIPS IT IS GOVERNMENT STYLE CAPTIALISM VERSUS ENTERPRISE

What Is Capitalism? "The chicken or the egg"

The best way I've found to justify capitalism is to compare it to other forms of socio-economic and political systems. To do this let's look at how the fruits of a chicken's labor are produced and disbursed under Nazism, Fascism, Socialism, Communism and finally Capitalism.

Nazism: This is where the government commandeers the hen before the eggs are hatched and raises the offspring as a perfect line. Only the bad eggs are given to the people.

> Fascism: This is where the government captures the eggs as they're laid, eats the yoke and gives the shells to the people.
>
> Socialism: This is where the people are given the hens. The eggs are laid according to the letter of the law and given to the people for one-half their wages in the form of Social Security taxes. The bad eggs are given back to the producers for recycling in accordance with environmental protection laws.
>
> Communism: This is where the hens are owned by the government. The eggs are commandeered by the

government for equal distribution to all. Only the average eggs are given to the people. The best eggs go to the Politburo. The good eggs go to the Olympic Team. If the annual quotas for production aren't met, the people are fed to the chickens.

Capitalism: This is where the people own the chickens. They buy the feed and risk their capital. The eggs are sold and the profits, if any, are taxed. The chickens are overworked and underpaid, but protected by unions. The unions guarantee collective bargaining, pensions, and equal opportunity for each and every chicken. The good eggs end up in the omelet's served to the law makers, the bad eggs are chastised by Russ Limbaugh and called Fascists, Nazis, Socialists and Communists.

In American parlance we do not have perfect capitalism when we have the government purchasing 75% of everything. You have a Monopsony (an Oligarchy). When you put the government in charge of being the purchaser of last resort for anything you have waste, loss of personal freedoms, misappropriation and average to below average results. (the impact of being average…the guy has a bare foot in the bucket of ice cold water and the other in a bucket of boiling hot water and on average he should feel great)…but in reality relegating everything to average is wasting away valuable resources on average to below average work ethic and guaranteed low quality.

In the final analysis, it's a question of which would you rather be: the chicken or the egg?

MONOPOSONY is where the chicken eats its own eggs:

1. The Red and the Blue are not accountable to problem resolution only their political disagreements on their selected social and fiscal issues.
    a. Public Servants have become Public Savants (savants may exhibit exceptional memory but have difficulty putting it to use. Savant skills are usually found in one or

more of five major areas: art, musical abilities, calendar calculation, Mathematics and spatial skills).
   b. Private Sector has become Private Slaves (taxpayers, workers and common folks).
2. A "yes-no" answer has been lost and honesty disregarded.
3. The dollar means more than moral character.
4. Financial and moral responsibility to constituencies is not a requirement for being elected.
5. The term "law maker" commits us to laws we do not need and cannot afford...it dilutes our freedoms according to the constitutional right to due process. This destroys the creativity of the "job makers" and individual freedoms.
6. Our democracy has out grown career politicians, unions and bureaucrats.
7. Fair representation means more than the class system that progressive or conservative policies have relegated to enterprising Americans.
8. Public sector and service union dominance over monetary and tax policy dumbs down the enterprising private sector...i.e., Americans' creative juices. The former Public Servants are now the Ruling Class.
9. The need for our Public and Private Governance to stand up for the Great American Enterprise and the Enterprising work ethic that is lost in the Oligarchy and the present socialized system.
10. The evolution of social systems predicts that socialism evolves into Communism where the Congress, Supreme Court and the Administration become the Politburo. After that is fascism and all personal freedoms are forever lost unless we have another American Revolution of 1776.

COOKING THE BOOKS COOKS OUR GOOSE

Government ignores the very rules that enterprise has to abide by... generally accepted accounting principles (GAAP) require that the debt for entitlements, pensions and accounts payable that apply to a particular fiscal period must be recorded and matched to revenues that have been earned...Government being on the cash basis intentionally accelerates collections of taxes (paying in estimates for the next period's (taxes) and defers expenditures as long as possible (unfunded but committed public sector pension costs, social security pension costs, and health care costs) creating the illusion that we are better off than we really are...the $16 trillion dollar deficit is really $100 trillion if GAAP was practiced. Why are we allowing our elected officials to mislead us into thinking that we are not as bad off as we really are?

COOKING THE ECONOMICS WITH INTEREST RATES

The Democratic Party Blue Economics; under "Keynesian" theory bigger government creates economic growth, cutting government spending hurts economic growth...Obama and his advisors are Keynesians...they believe that government spending creates infrastructure jobs and grows the economy...that using the Federal Reserve Banking System to set exchange interest rates controls inflation and increasing taxes to balance the growth of the Federal Budget controls the American economy.

The Republican Party Red Economics; under "trickle down" economic theory increasing taxes hurts economic growth...Reagan and his advisors were trickle down advocates...they and current conservation Republicans believe that cutting taxes creates jobs and grows the economy by giving entrepreneurs, small businesses and risk takers more capital to create jobs and grows the economy....however, in practice they promote continued growth of Big Government and as a byproduct want to cut acceptable entitlements and use lawmaking and punitive regulations to further control.

COOLING THE DEBT AND HEATING UP THE ECONOMY

The American Enterprise Party Economic formula = smaller government and elimination of the new entitlements induces profitable business enterprise...by downsizing government, privatizing regulatory agencies and economizing the cost of Government creates the dynamics of enterprise which are jobs, jobs, jobs, profits, taxable income and GNP growth. Through reduced Government overhead, capital development thrives, the deficits are eliminated, national debt is paid down and America's needed entitlements are intact.

> The War on Debt Economics formula = mobilized workers, focused objectives, measurable goals, adequate financing for the duration, disciplined approach to work, flexible work hours, decks cleared of obstacles to mission (over regulation), measurable results…examples WWI and WWII created economic growth while the subsequent wars were not motivated by nationalism…because of the limitations put on the reason for the missions i.e., no definable outcome and no resulting growth in income.

So let's mobilize the Constitution…use the Enterprise structure, composition and makeup of America to start a new form of Government Enterprise…use the basic constitutional law in a socially organized third party…to do as the founding fathers pointed out, Enterprise and Capital are required, both human and monetary… so downsizing Government, economizing natural resources, recapitalizing America's Enterprise by using investment incentives, for those who have high net worth, to capitalize small businesses, entrepreneurial initiatives and funding risk takers is the essence of this book.

The real answers to great questions are below the obvious and above conventional wisdom, as Michael Crichton said, "Conventional wisdom is invariably out of date. Because in the time it has taken to become conventional wisdom, and become what everyone believes to be true, the world has moved on. Conventional wisdom is a remnant of the past".

Conventional wisdom and past experience demonstrates that a third political party cannot win…until now…10 reasons why we need an effective third party alternative that is functional in controlling the runaway wasteful cost of Government:

It comes down to pursuing positive solutions to negative externalities, as defined in Super Freakonomics, by Steven Levitt and Stephen

Dubner ...what is an externality? "It's what happens when someone takes an action but someone else, without agreeing, pays some or all the costs of this action. An externality is an economic version of taxation without representation. The Greenhouse gasses thought to be responsible for global warming are primarily externalities since each of us are generating some by-products we are not paying for"... for example if we are obese and don't pay for our health care costs... if we are retired we are not paying for our health benefits...we are not internalizing the cost and when we aren't compelled to pay the full cost of our actions, we have little incentive to change our behavior. "Today, people are being asked to change their behavior not out to self-interest but rather out of selflessness".

"Not all externalities are negative". A positive externality is when we pay for public education and have no kids in school. That's why we have entitlements...to positively share in the cost of positive externalities. In their first book, Freakonomics the authors establish that "moral incentives are the way we would like things to be and economic incentives are the way things are"...so a third party political alternative is a needed economic incentive to have the common good internalize (fund through taxation) the positive entitlement externalities for the Greater Good of the American Enterprise. But the taxation must be for that purpose...not the irrational expansion of the Public Sector.

THE REST OF THE STORY

Michael Creighton, bestselling author wrote a book entitled "Fear Factor" where he is quoted as saying that fear is used as tactic for forcing political agendas on the masses ... in the best-selling novel by Yann Martel, is a magical adventure **story** centering on **Pi** Patel, the precocious son of a zoo keeper that establishes that fear is the only thing fatal to life. So fear is used incessantly by politicians, bureaucrats and media to make us comply with their initiatives, opinions and issues; all the while distracting us from the reality of fairness.

For example: our negative financial condition is caused by entitlements...so we have to stop our spending spree on those fixed costs even though we will hurt them. This abstract thinking is forgetting what is right and wrong. First of all Social Security and Medicare do not belong to the Government and Medicaid is a safety net paid for by the taxpayers for that purpose...these are trust funds belonging to the beneficiaries. To deprive them of entitled benefits is illegal and should not be touched for the reasons they are being dissipated...loans to the General Fund, purchase of Treasury Notes, payment of interest on national debt, rationing of the funds for care to others, etc. We do not have the legal right to impound these entitlements. We don't need Entitlement Reform we need Government Reform.

We need to destroy the MONOPSONY before it destroys us.

For example the bureaucracy has grown out of control at every level. Iowa has 189 committees, boards and subcommittees using party line volunteer patronage positions to control opposition. Illinois the worst run State in the Union has 355 patronage barnacles hanging us with a debt of 80 billion dollars in debt. Fort Worth has 45 standing committees. Total size of the paid employees of Government at all levels is 19.7 million and rising with a $1 trillion annual payroll and $25 trillion in unfunded pension costs. Total Federal debt of $125 trillion dollars if all obligations were on the books.

For example we need and can reduce spending on the new entitlements (unemployment, workers' comp, food stamps, public pensions, disability, etc.) that have not been entrusted to the Government. They are diluting the work ethic and forcing businesses to pay expenses that are not related to producing products, profits and taxes...Government should be funding these entitlements out of American style Enterprise increases in the GNP and GDP if at all.

Serving the Greater Good—Through an Enterprise Model

The foundation of American democracy is the pursuit of the greater good. As a country, we pursue what is good for most of the people most of the time. But that is not our approach for the care of our elderly. Of the 313 million people in America, seventy-seven million are baby boomers. In the next ten years, a staggering majority of them will turn sixty. Even though it would be for the greater good of America, there are no provisions for taking care of these aging lives.

There are only time bombs:

- Currently, there are 3.2 million falls per year among the elderly in nursing homes. There will be eighty million per year when the baby boomers come of nursing-home age.
- On the average, baby boomers will have four to five chronic illnesses by the time they are sixty-five—that equates to 350 million chronic conditions.
- Seventy-seven million families will be affected by the disabilities and chronic conditions imposed on them by aging baby boomers.
- Seventy-seven million households are not equipped and never will be to handle chronic illnesses and dependent lives.
- About $77 trillion will be imposed annually on the budgets of state and federal governments to care for the aging boomers.
- Seventy-seven million voters will be enraged by the lack of preparation for and health-care coverage for the greater good.
- Those same seventy-seven million voters, with an average yearly spending of fifty thousand that adds up to $3.86 trillion, do *not* want to spend their money on the current health care system. They would rather invest in health preservation than in health maintenance.
- The forty-six million uninsured will become one hundred million as the baby boomers become of retirement age and unemployed.
- There are currently 1.7 million nursing home patients in sixteen thousand nursing homes and four million assisted-living residents in twenty-three thousand assisted-living facilities.

We will need seventeen times as many nursing homes and eighteen times as many assisted-living facilities to handle the seventy-seven million baby boomers in a supportive setting.
- One million physicians, 2.4 million nurses, four thousand five hundred hospitals, sixteen thousand nursing homes, and 6.4 million other health professionals cannot handle the needs of seventy-seven million aging baby boomers who want their share of the health-care dollars. Making the radical change from health maintenance to prevention and health preservation would serve the greater good and make more Medicare money available.

On top of these time bombs, we have seventy-seven million high expectations. If we are expecting these seventy-seven million baby boomers to just accept nursing homes and assisted living as they are, think again. They tend to be dependent on others for their approach to health care and generally are not staying healthy, nor are they schooled in preserving their health and do not want to pay more for preventing poor health. Compounding this, their health-care providers are not schooled in detecting cause or in pursuing measurable outcomes. But they are paid regardless of results.

THE ENTERPRISE MODEL—A NEW PARADIGM

Sharon Rhoads, wife of the author, whose mother, Dorotha C. White, for whom the Dorotha C. White Foundation (*www.dcwhitefoundation.org*) was formed, died of abuse and neglect in a nursing home. It was not of her choosing, and we feel guilty for putting her there. Due to circumstances similar to most families, there was no other alternative. Sharon and I are in the business of assisting nursing homes to improve their programming and provide the companionship, emotional counseling, socialization, and spiritual services that are so direly needed. With the "adopt a patient program," we are dedicated to avoiding occurrences that befell Dorotha.

Across America, we adopt highways, foreign-born babies, laws, domestic-born babies, foster children, etc. All this effort is to exercise the heart of a free society, which is to give all human beings a chance at life liberty and the pursuit of happiness. We need to *restore elderpride* for the sake of ourselves as we all will need quality of care for our quality-of-life wishes. Quality of life (QOL) differs from quality of care (QOC) since QOL is outcome-driven and QOC is income-driven. QOL incentive is focused on restorative services and discharge, and QOC is focused on treatment and medications for generating revenues. QOL incorporates the economic incentives of enterprise since it pays for results (deductive processes—destination is holistic journey) not just action (inductive processes—destination is a procedure) and for outcome, not just income.

Where this dichotomy of philosophy seems to be best exemplified is at the choke hold government has on our nursing homes. The resulting institutionalization of the elderly is pandemic and will get much worse with the aging of the baby boomers. I am not an advocate of dumping them back into the community that is not capable or ready to take on such a huge responsibility. My philosophy is that the nursing homes are not homes for the elderly. They are called such, and society accepts it as the only alternative. I propose there is another alternative:

1. QOL recognizes that skilled-nursing care is not home care; it is transitional care.
2. QOL replaces the medical model practiced by physicians, hospitals, and nursing homes with the restorative model.
3. QOL encourages community involvement in making the transition.
4. QOL mandate a reimbursement system that rewards outcomes that improve and restore function.
5. QOL sets up community-based programs that assist in the restoration of the elderly back into the community-based services; "adopt a patient" is that kind of involvement that is needed.
6. QOL requires that technology be utilized for processing the outcome-driven assessment of need, delivery of services, and the evaluation of outcome justifying the price, cost, and return-on-investment formula.

QOL embraces the body, the mind, the heart, and the spirit. This is where the Adopt a Nursing Home Patient Program is critical. Missing in most all nursing homes is the companionship factor, the emotional uplift factor, the socializing factor, and the spiritual factor. Why? Because the staff is not organized to deliver holistic care. It is given lip service at best. We have done studies, and literally none of the nursing homes are providing psycho/social programming because they are not being paid for it. This is an alarming fact.

To solve this will take the effort of the community, the politicians, the clinicians, the providers, and the families. Under our Adopt a Nursing Home Patient, we are dealing with all four factors:

- Companionship—a visit by a real person who is interested in the patient's feelings, needs, problems, and hopes that will create healing that is not medicinal.
- Emotions—writing a letter to a patient who does not receive mail revitalizes the humanity of knowing someone cares.
- Socialization—currently the patients are grouped around TVs in wheelchairs with no social stimulation. Why not take a patient to a movie outside the facility and go out to eat and go to the ballgame?
- Spiritual stimulation—church can be brought to the patient, or the patient can be taken to church. It takes someone doing it.

The foundation will obtain authorization from the provider, the family, and the State regulators to provide the "adoption of a patient" by a community volunteer to provide the companionship, emotional involvement, socialization, and spiritual contact for those who need it, want it, and will sign an approval for it.

Why will the provider of care agree to this? The foundation, on its website, will provide free advertising for those providers implementing the "adopt a patient" program. The facility must assist in screening the volunteers coming into their facility and measure the effectiveness of the program. The foundation will rate the facility using six-star criteria before allowing them to participate in the program:

* First star is for companionship through the use of the "adopt a patient" program.
* Second star is for environment cleanliness: no odors, plenty of light, live plants, pets, etc.
* Third star is for efficient and productive staffing: staff organized in teams to provide restorative services and able to show improvements in functioning.
* Fourth star is for social programs: for example, reading groups, current-events groups, storytelling groups, discussion groups geared to disease process, etc.
* Fifth star is for psychological counseling programs use of group therapies, reducing prescriptions as the alternative to treatment, and replacing it with more exercise and better nutritional alternatives.
* Sixth star is for spiritual involvement of the community churches by allowing the patients to come to outside services.

The foundation rating as a six-star facility will get the Dorotha C. White Foundation certification as a flagship facility. A five-star facility will get the DCW Foundation certification as an excellent facility. A four-star rating will get the certification as a good facility. Any facility under the four stars will not be allowed to participate in the "adopt a patient" program.

Why will the family of the patient agree to this? Studies have shown that visitation in nursing homes is at an all-time low due to odors, depressive surroundings, seeing the aging process as discouraging, observing the low esteem of the workers, insensitive providers, state and federal enforcement tactics, etc. We believe that the "adopt a patient" program can bring positive forces to bear volunteerism, benevolence, free services for cleaning and keeping the facility up, community services brought to the patient rather than vice versa. We believe the families are not visiting due to time restraints and families to raise as well. So why not help them out and set an example that companionship makes a big difference in the patients will to live.

Why would the state and federal regulators welcome this program? The goal of every surveyor I ever met was to improve the quality of life of those in nursing homes. Since it is not happening on a consistent basis and they know it, they will welcome it. And in fact, many agencies are paying for most of these services in their Medicaid-rate setting and not getting it. We all can see that the enforcement tactics do not work.

Why would a person in a community that has no loved one in a facility agree to do this? Why do we have people adopting foreign orphans, domestic foster children, keeping a highway clean, helping the elderly do their shopping, and helping the elderly stay warm or cool in inclement weather? Americans, in fact, do have a big heart when they know there is a need. In nursing homes, the term *eldercide* has been coined by the foundation because the elderly are systematically institutionalized against their will and kept there until they die a lonely and scarred death. Elder pride is the goal of the foundation accomplished by adopting patients and eliciting outsiders to assist in the paradigm shift to a true quality of life on the inside.

THE SENATE
By: Jerry Rhoads

They sit behind
Dappled desks
On seats of power

Surrounded by
The tides of a deep heritage
Of Congress the balance of power

With a constitution
And a declaration of independence
Supporting this power

The statues stand
In buildings of stature
And Magnitude

In testimony to
How deep the American
Blood flows

Flowing from strong
Dedicated men believing
In sovereign principles

With all others asked to be
As strong
But can they be

Can they believe
As deeply
As America's blood flows

Are they more than
Themselves
Or just a picture

Of their ego
The phantoms of the Senate
Behind dappled desks

Lining the marbled halls
The seats of power
Revered by shallow men

Distained by the weakling
Loved by idealists
Born from a belief in good fortune

A vein of gold
Inlaid upon a fallow land
Signifying the American heritage

A vein of obscurity
A vein of red, white and blue blood
Flowing from the hearts of millions

Holding their leaders up to the light
To see if their ideals
Their principles, with humility, prevail

Tossing away those that are
Transparent and too flexible
To be the levy, and the strength

To be our next heritage
The ides of a deep bondage
From the words of Gettysburg

To the dark shadow of Hiroshima
And the conquest of inner space
Far deeper than outer space

Senator, senator, hearken
Hear this message or
Perish from the seat of power

You are not sacred
You are not above principle
You are only a human flower

Rooted in responsibility
To pledge allegiance
To our heritage and we empower

To you our Republic
For which it stands
One nation indivisible under God

With liberty and justice for all
So do not let the
Great American Enterprise Fall

SUMMARY OF ENTERPRISE MODEL COMPONENTS
(shifts the paradigm from fee for treatment to fee for outcome):

Mutual insurance companies collect the premiums using health profiles of its individual shareholders. It matches premiums to that profile.

Each individual manages their own expenditures under a defined benefit formula.

Providers are paid on a QOL episodic basis for their standard cost for that episode requiring cost accounting and standard costing and pricing as defined in their contract with the mutual insurance company. Continuums of care consolidation will be encouraged to make the enterprise more efficient and effective.

- Physicians are paid for predetermined procedures based on outcome criteria for recovery, recuperation, rehabilitation, and restoration of the full person (the definition of outcome).
- Hospitals are paid for predetermined procedures based on outcome criteria for recovery, recuperation, rehabilitation, and restoration of the full person (the definition of outcome).
- Nursing homes are paid for predetermined procedures based on outcome criteria for recovery, recuperation, rehabilitation, and restoration of the full person (the definition of outcome).
- Assisted-living homes are paid for predetermined procedures based on outcome criteria for recovery, recuperation, rehabilitation, and restoration of the full person (the definition of outcome).
- Home-care agencies are paid for predetermined procedures based on outcome criteria for recovery, recuperation, rehabilitation, and restoration of the full person (the definition of outcome).
- Hospice agencies are paid for predetermined procedures based on outcome criteria for recovery, recuperation, rehabilitation, and restoration of the full person (the definition of outcome).

See Jerry Rhoads's books for the basis of standard costing and pricing formulas for health care.

THE LAST CHAPTER

We have been forced to sell the two Iowa facilities. Closing will take place in a few days. To let us know we are the arch enemy of the Monopsony we have had surveyors in both facilities on self-reports and complaints (that I consider violation of my fifth-amendment rights to due process) alleging improper supervision of care and allowing patients to escape. These carry harsh civil money penalties and admission hold remedies. Hopefully, the new owners know better how to deal with the Monopsony.

As victims of the Biggest Bully's ire and Catch 23's violation of our fifth-amendment rights I end this book with the foibles of the Iowa "Gotcha System" that Governor Branstad stated he did not want. First of all there were no changes in the tactics or staff after he made Rod Roberts, a former legislator, the Director. The Governors are the keepers of the Monopsony Board and with fear and threats of jail time they will manage to kill the enterprise goose called American ingenuity ... our experience proves that.

Monopsony tactics using the "Gotcha System" violates Human Rights:

It is an example of the American Government enforcement unfettered that curtails Human Rights to due process of law when Catch 23 exists. It destroys Human Dignity, Human initiative, Human problem solving, Human creativity, Human freedoms. The very allegations our Government make against the "Axis of Evil" and Ferguson, Brown, Rodney King, etc.

1. Providers have no rights to due process of law. The Administrative Procedures Act that the State is to follow is ignored allowing arbitrary and capricious enforcement tactics while the Department of Inspections and Appeals is immune from lawsuit.

2. The smaller the provider the more the F-tags (notification of a violation of the minimum standards of care) and the harsher the penalties doled out. Family owned nursing homes are a thing of the past ... oh, those mom pops don't have the ability to run a health care business.
3. The larger the chain provider the fewer the F-tags and the more the politicians get in PAC money.
4. The trade associations lobby for more money and do not tug on the Biggest Bully's cape.
5. The big brother Monopsony (Department of Health and Human Services) utilizes its Gestapo CMS and OIG teams to threaten and cohere the provider associations, chains and independents with rules and regulations that are based in criminal law not civil law so they can use fear as their most egregious tactic. They infer that every provider is committing fraud and abuse and are guilty until proven innocent (what happened to the fifth-amendment?).
6. Reimbursement was initially to be cost plus but that gave way to cost minus when the Monopsony found out it could not pay its bills. This resulted in changes in the application of the Medicare trust funds that violated Federal law ... the Congress changed the way they pay not what they pay for because that would take a change in the Medicare law. So instead of breaking the law they finagled the payment from retrospective to prospective forcing the providers to be paid on input units not output units of service. Now there is no connection between Provider income and outcome. The next step removes the Monopsony's accountability to pay for quality and moves it to a quantity based system called capitation.
7. Under the Obama Monopsony a person's age will dictate the premiums and services. The younger are expected to pay more because they are healthy and the older will get less and less services because the young cannot afford to pay for chronic illnesses, obesity and senility. Eventually the Monopsony will deny claims due to preexisting chronic illnesses and cap the amount that will be covered at all. The promise to cover everyone for everything and it will not cost one dime will

haunt those lawmakers who passed the bill without reading it or representing their constituents.
8. Under the Obama Monopsony Game more will be spent on FBI, IRS, OIG enforcement (1 trillion dollars over the first 10 years) and (demonstration projects granted to Universities to prove what CMS has already decided (1 trillion dollars over the first 10 years) than the needs of the Baby Boomers. President Obama was right when he said it won't cost one dime ... more like a zillion dimes. Now we are talking Google dollars and Monopsony taxes. If our foreign policy doesn't bankrupt us our Monopsony Game will.

PS: I just got off the phone with the buyer and attorneys and the deal is about to fall through. We received untimely minor self-reported "gotcha" deficiencies that could stop the closing. So the beat goes on and on and on and on until we as a country realize that most human beings are not important as we march to the tune of our own version of Animal Farm where some people are more equal than others.

When the sale of the facilities is finally closed we admit we lost every battle with the Monopsony. But the war goes on. Shari and I plan to form a lobby proposing legislation to change the paradigm from Government run health care to –

1. Collaboration with the private sector on amending Obama Care to an Enterprise driven, outcome based system.
2. Privatization of the payment system based on individualized care plans and economic incentives based on positive outcomes.
3. Funding through a combination of taxation and withholding accounts for employed Americans with a safety net for the elderly and indigent Americans.
4. Retaining Medicare for the elderly safety net and Medicaid for the unemployed safety net. This will be administered by each State's Mutually owned private insurance companies.

AFTERWORD

As an example of Government and Private businesses collaborating is the very successful Medisave system in Singapore. An Asian country of 4 million.

The author's SHIFT the paradigm system is similar to this Singapore Healthcare System that is the most cost effective and efficient and quality driven solution in the world today. They are number 1 in quality and number 1 in lowest cost per capita.

The system was developed by Private business and Government working in collaboration.

Their Stated Philosophy:

The Ministry of Health believes in ensuring **quality and affordable basic medical services** for all.

At the same time, the Ministry promotes **healthy living** and **preventive health programs** as well as maintains **high standards of living, clean water and hygiene** to achieve better health for all.

Structure and Budget

Singapore's healthcare system is designed to ensure that everyone has access to different levels of healthcare in a timely, cost-effective and seamless manner.

Healthcare Services and Facilities

Healthcare services are accessible through a wide network of primary, acute and step-down care providers. *More*

Healthcare Regulation

The Ministry of Health and its statutory boards regulate both the public and private providers of healthcare in Singapore.

Quality and Innovation

To ensure that patients are treated safely with good healthcare standards, the Ministry strives to promote better quality and innovation through various initiatives.

Schemes & Subsidies

An introduction to the healthcare system in Singapore.

Medisave, introduced in April 1984, is a national medical savings scheme which helps individuals put aside part of their income into their Medisave Accounts to meet their future personal or immediate family's hospitalization, day surgery and certain outpatient expenses. Find out more about Medisave.

MediShield, introduced in 1990, is a low cost catastrophic illness insurance scheme. It is designed to help members meet the medical expenses from major or prolonged illnesses from which their Medisave balance would not be sufficient to cover. MediShield operates on a co-payment and deductible system to avoid the problems associated with first-dollar, comprehensive insurance. The premiums for MediShield is payable by Medisave.

Medifund is an endowment fund set up by the Government in April 1993 to help needy Singaporeans who are unable to pay for their medical expenses. This fund acts as a safety net for those who cannot afford the subsidized bill charges despite Medisave and MediShield coverage. Medifund was established with an initial capital of S$200 million and capital injections will be made when budget surpluses are available. The capital sum currently stands at S$1.7 billion. The interest income from this capital sum are being utilized to finance the needy.

ElderShield, introduced in September 2002, is an affordable severe disability insurance scheme designed to help Singaporeans meet with expenses incurred in the event of severe disability. ElderShield premiums can be paid with Medisave or cash.

Other subsidy schemes

The Interim Disability Assistance Programme for the Elderly (IDAPE) scheme provides financial help to need and disabled Singaporeans, who were not eligible to join ElderShield due to their age and pre-existing conditions.

The Community Health Assist Scheme (CHAS) is one of the Ministry of Health (MOH)'s programs to help provide accessible and affordable medical and dental care to Singapore Citizens.

Patients receive drug subsidies based on their paying status and the scheme under which the drug is covered (e.g. Standard Drug List, Medication Assistance Fund, inpatient drug subsidy, etc). Some drugs are subsidized only for specific clinical indications.

The Caregivers Training Grant (CTG) provides caregivers with an annual grant of $200 for each care dependent to attend AIC's pre-approved training programs. It aims to build the caregiver's capabilities in caring for the physical, social and emotional needs of the care recipients.

What are the metrics that prove Singapore's health care system is working better than any other approach in the world. Singapore's life expectancy is superior:

Nation Life Expectancy

- Singapore 82
- Australia 81.5
- Canada 81.2
- Japan 81
- France 80.5

- Sweden 80.5
- Switzerland 80.5
- Germany 79.5
- United Kingdom 78.5
- USA 78

Singapore's costs as a percent of GNP is superior to America.

Health Expenditures
Nation % of GDP

- USA 16%
- Singapore 3.25%
- Canada 9%
- Japan 8%
- Germany 10%
- United Kingdom 8%

Government share of the spending is reduced to a manageable level and accomplishing the objective of having a public option and a single payer system using the savings accounts administered by the Government but the spending decisions left with the individuals. The savings accounts are the backbone for this Enterprise Model of health care because it introduces supply and demand and competition to the equation. This does not occur in America where someone else is responsible for making the buying and paying decisions. Where an insurance company or the Government pays the bill the individual does not internalize the necessity to stay fit and practice wellness habits. My Proposed SHIFT SYSTEM (Self-Health Insurance Funding Trust) embodies the Enterprise Model and will produce the same results that are being demonstrated in Singapore.

Ironically, the Singapore system sounds vaguely familiar. Our original social security and Medicare Great Society programs were designed to collaborate between government and private sectors for many of the Singapore principles. Then Congress interfered making them no longer trust funds but availability for loans to the general fund borrowing for fighting wars and paying debt service. Even though technically illegal the social security and Medicare funds no longer exist as Trust Funds. Monopsony at work again destroys intent and purpose.

EXHIBIT A

The Real Victims of the Monopsony

LTC Insurance Is a Victim of the Monopsony

Monopsony ... a market situation in which there is only one buyer. Unless we break it up it will break us down. In the final analysis the following is an example of what the implications are:

In an article by James Berklan, editor of McKnight's daily news report, laments the demise of long term care insurance.

"There is a memorable scene in the movie "Forrest Gump" when Lt. Dan chews out the well-intentioned title soldier for saluting him while the enemy is likely watching. The implication is that if you want to strike a crushing blow to something, you take out its leader.

Call it cutting off the head of the snake, taking out the top guy or whatever you want. Not only does eliminating a leader erase a primary means of getting direction, it also kills morale.

That's what I pondered Tuesday when I saw the bad news about long-term care insurer Genworth Financial. It is the largest U.S. seller of long-term care insurance and a holdout among the many large insurers that once sold LTC policies.

Gone, exiting the market or decreasing exposure are names like, MetLife, Unum and Hancock. But Genworth, despite, has always remained.

Capturing more than one-third of the long-term care insurance market, Genworth would be the one to stick it out. Genworth was the stalwart. (OK, it announced it would have to get tougher about bottom line considerations. Annual premium increases, lesser likelihood of payouts down the road, and vanishing inflation hedges. But No. 1 would be marching on.)

Now, however, it might be time to yell, "Run, Forrest, run!"

Cracks that began to show, if not earlier, have made Genworth's long-term care business worthless. At least that's at Macquarie Group Ltd. and Keefe, Bruyette and Woods.

On Monday, in fact, one of the analysts called for the LTC to close up shop.

Seems that recovery efforts attempted by Genworth CEO Tom McInerney are having trouble gaining traction. A third-quarter loss of $844 million was announced last week, triggering a 40% drop in stock value. This, in the wake of raising premiums and cutting future policy benefits. Not exactly the stuff of inspiration."

The Author's underlying point is what Monopsony's do they force out competition and destroy initiative. As Obama Monopsony Care prevails the private enterprise sector will be forced out and we will be stuck with VA care. Solution: breakup the Monopsony by privatizing health care before it cuts the head off the snake and eventually tells all of us "sorry you are too old to be admitted to the hospital … it is too costly to keep you alive … you're half dead anyway". The Monopsony calls this end of life care.

Providers Are Victims of the Monopsony Game

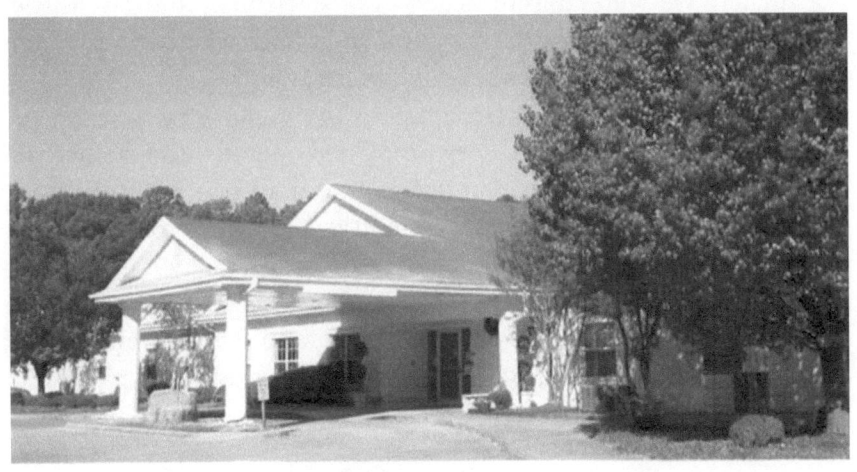

LITTLE ROCK – VICTIM #1

The Rhoads' purchased this 139 bed facility in November 2009. It was troubled and was going to be closed. In eighteen months we invested over $500,000 to renovate and change the culture from a warehouse for nursing home patients to a care house for human being needing health care services.

Victimized: Within two and one half months of taking over the facility the State surveyors managed to turn a minor injury in the transport van into an Immediate Jeopardy violation (patient unfastened his seat belt and fell). This ultimately prevented us from keeping the facility.

After their enforcement action, they forced us to reapply for our Medicare and Medicaid certification, or be shut down. Then put a hold on admissions until the surveyors gave us a clean bill of health. This cost us over $1 million dollars in revenue that we had to borrow from the bank.

This arbitrary and capricious act reduced the sales price of the nursing home from $7,600,000 to $4,650,000 and we were sued by the builder for $2,700,000 the amount it took to emerge from special focus and get a new provider numbers from Medicare and Medicaid. Fortunately we were able to negotiate a settlement and left Little Rock behind to an operator that put it right back where it was when we took it over. A warehouse for indigent patients.

During the eighteen months we owned and operated the facility we remodeled the exterior and interior, removed all odors, turned over all of the staff and implemented restorative care. This enabled us to move from number 13 in quality to number 3 as the choice of the surrounding hospital discharge planners. Our Medicare program was the best in the city and the value to the community was enhanced. The true measure of quality.

> "This is the cleanest, nicest looking nursing home I have ever been in and the lunch was scrumptious. You've made such difference here."
>
> *Unsolicited remarks from*
> *Mike Mitchell, attorney at law.*

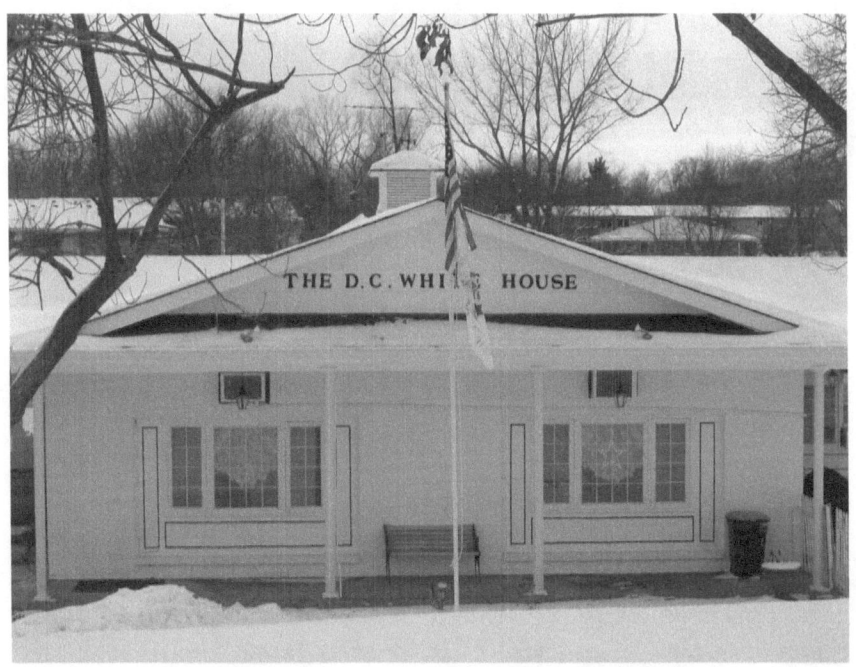

MUSCATINE – VICTIM #2

The Rhoads' purchased this 100 bed facility in September 2009. It was troubled and was going to be closed. In eighteen months we invested over $500,000 to renovate and change the culture from a warehouse for nursing home patients to a care house for human being needing health care services.

Victimized: Within days of closing the sale of our two Iowa nursing homes, caused by the enforcement actions taken against us, the Surveyors' managed to turn a minor incident with a troubled Alzheimer's patient into an Immediate Jeopardy violation that effectively prevented us from closing the sale of the facilities.

After the State's enforcement action, resulting in $8,000 per day in civil money penalties and fines for 41 days or a total of $328,000 of civil money penalties, CMS put a hold on our admissions till the surveyors gave us a clean bill of health.

This arbitrary and capricious act reduced the contracted sales price of the two nursing homes from $8,500,000 to $5,850,000 that in essence bankrupted the our small businesses.

We had to put our banks and our vendors on a payment plan until we could go back to the marketplace to solicit another buyer at a reduced price.

To date we are still trying to get out of this crazy business that is now being dominated by the Monopsony and its large conglomerates managing real estate investments for incomes not quality patient outcomes.

During the five and one half years we owned and operated the Muscatine facility we remodeled the exterior and interior, removed all odors, turned over 90% of the staff and implemented restorative care. This enabled us to discharge 57% of our admissions back into the community ... unheard of in nursing home circles. The true measure of quality.

> *"I never make it a point to brag on a facility I tour but I have to tell you I am amazed by your staff ... they are friendly, smile, and every room is clean, organized with all the beds made. Everyone I talk to loves this place."*
>
> **Unsolicited comments by**
> Judy a volunteer Ombudsman.

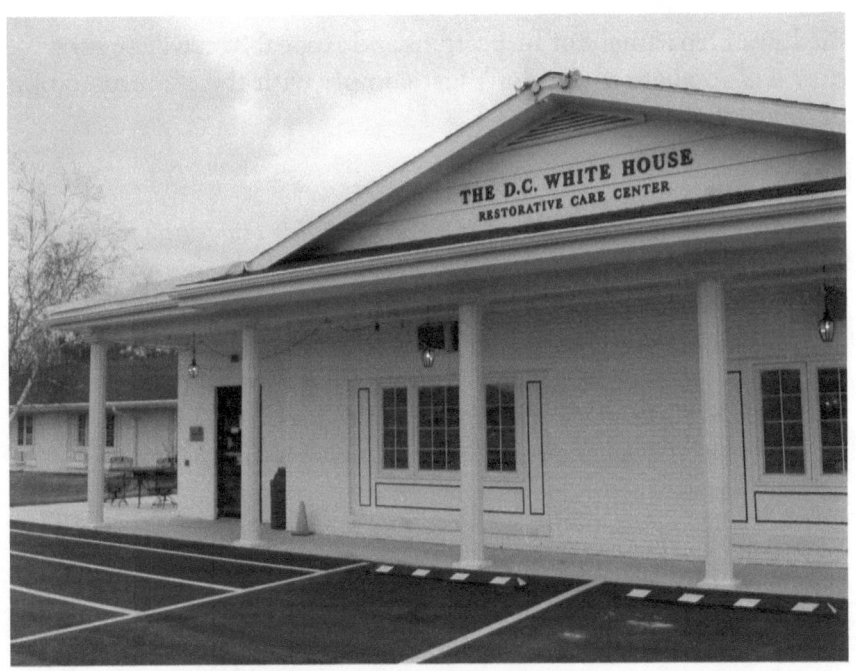

WASHINGTON – VICTIM #3

The Rhoads' purchased this 125 bed facility in October 2011. It was troubled and was going to be closed. In thirty eight months we invested over $500,000 to renovate and change the culture from a warehouse for nursing home patients to a care house for human being needing health care services.

During the three and one half years we owned and operated the Washington facility we remodeled the exterior and interior, removed all odors, turned over 90% of the staff and implemented restorative care. Even though we were targeted by the Monopsony we discharged more and more of our patients back home ... the true measure of quality.

Victimized: Within two and one half months after acquiring the facility State surveyors managed to turn an incident in the Alzheimer's unit into a Special Focus violation that cost us $100,000 in fines, $100,000 in legal fees, that eventually forced us to sell our nursing homes and scuttle our original goals. We were warned that if we fight the Iowa Department of Inspections and Appeals you will be sorry ... they will retaliate if you don't just comply with their interpretation of minor violations.

> *"I was told this facility is terrible before I came here. Of course this came from people in the community that have never been here and believe what they read in the newspaper. And I was dreading having to come here. But now that I am here I cannot believe how there is no foul odor, it is extremely clean. It looks good and in my opinion the detractors should come here before they judge you by the surveys posted by the State on the internet."*
>
> **Unsolicited evaluation by**
> Dave a new volunteer Ombudsman.

SUMMARY

Our original plan was to acquire troubled skilled nursing facilities, modernize them, computerize them, scour them, change the culture to that of restoring patients for discharge and improve the quality of life of those that have to stay. Admirable and thought to be profitable for all involved.

This entailed utilizing the Caregiver Management system of software and operational management tools. Our care planning system is the platform for assigning the workload to the staff, organize the workflow, cost the labor and ancillaries, and restorative programming for clinical and social services. With the two models we were building in Iowa we had plans of acquiring other rural facilities and setting up a franchise business where the owner would be on site every day promoting accountability with authority so the quality of care and life would be controlled locally not corporately.

All of these plans were brought crashing down with the punitive interventions of the Department of Inspections and Appeals. The Monopsony destroys everything under it.

Is this a scenario of bad luck, poor management, bad care or punitive enforcement and retaliation. It hurt the three communities, the 300 staff, 225 patients, 225 families and future of those facilities. After you have read this far make you own conclusion ... but consider the fact that every good deed gets punished and this set of circumstances did not make the dramatic turn around and difference in the care the Rhoads family made the difference ... they made the conversions of bad management, bad care and bad luck into modernized and quality of life operations that enabled them to sell the facilities and come out of bankruptcy in spite of the regulators. It is their plan to forget the battles but continue the war on the Monopsony.

If We Lose
The Monopsony Game

- Federal spending will escalate as it becomes the purchaser of last resort.
- 40,000 laws passed per year across America.
- Taxes on every commodity and service.
- Small businesses disappear as conglomerates grow.
- Leadership in the world will continue to decline.

If We Win
The Monopsony Game

- Privatize half of Government.
- Repeal 10 laws for every law passed.
- Rebase taxes on outcome not income.
- Enterprise will thrive.
- Leadership in the world guaranteed.

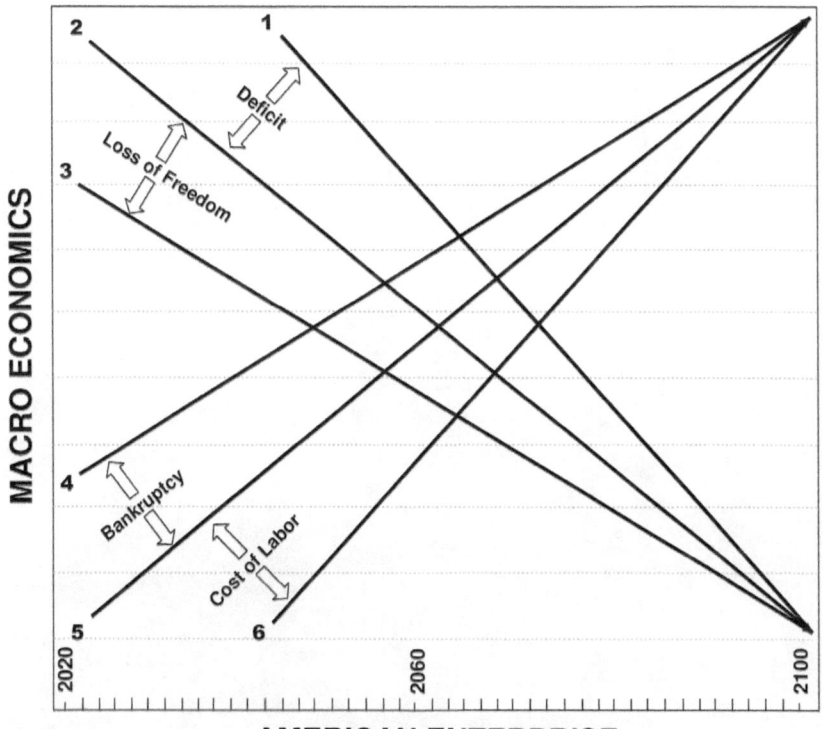

Winning The Monopsony Game:

This Monopsony Game can be won, if and when the voters decide to slow the growth of government; control taxation; remove unneeded laws that produce more resources for wage growth for the working Americans; improve small business employee's morale; and allow for the benefits of competition, such as creativity, technology and profitability. Thereby reducing the deficits and labor costs, while getting rid of laws that inhibit small business and GNP growth and solidifying America's position of economic leadership in the world, would create a "Win-Win" for everyone.

LEGEND

1 —— Size of Government
2 —— Taxes
3 —— Laws
4 —— Competition
5 —— GNP Growth
6 —— Work Ethic

INDEX

A

AAC (All-American Care), 82, 97, 102–3, 137, 153, 156, 180, 194, 196–97, 212
abuse, 59, 61–63, 109, 139, 150, 152–53, 163, 165–66, 170, 190, 237
abuse of discretion, 56–57, 139–40
accommodations, 27–28
ACOs (accountable care organizations), 6, 86–87, 89
acuity, 110
adjudicators, 192
Administrative Procedure Act, 44, 57, 82, 102–3, 136, 139, 156–57, 161
administrative remedies, 43–44
admissions, 50, 64, 76–79, 81, 108–9, 132, 138, 154–58, 160, 163, 173, 175–76, 179, 195, 201, 205–6, 220, 246, 255, 257–58
  new, 45, 101, 143, 145, 163
adopt-a-patient program, 237, 239–40
Aetna, 14, 73–74
Affordable Golf Club Act, 53
Alexian Brothers, 169
allegations, 37, 44, 46, 55, 61, 76, 78, 82, 101, 105, 109, 134, 136, 138–39, 143, 147–48, 150–54, 156–57, 161, 165, 174, 176, 205–7, 211–12, 220
ALOS (average length of stay), 61

Alzheimer's, 103, 124, 166, 192, 204, 213
Ambassador Club, 185–86
American businesses, 63, 113
American economy, 113, 232
American Health Care Association, 82, 273
ancillaries, 27, 29, 31, 261
annual survey, 77, 118, 149, 226
appeal rights, 43, 50, 59, 145–46, 212
Award for Quality Care in Health Care Facilities, 198, 201

B

baby boomers, 13, 71, 75, 112, 236–38, 248
Bianchi (doctor), 166–67, 169, 172
biggest bully, 8, 34, 37, 45, 50, 82
biggest problem, 59
Bigol (doctor), 163, 166, 169
blood thinners, 132, 184
Blue Cross, 72, 113, 190
Branstad (governor), 76, 107, 198–200, 246
Brennan, Paula, 163–64, 166, 171
bully pulpit, 34, 37
BUN (Blood Urea Nitrogen), 164
business, 6, 10, 14, 17–18, 23, 27, 29, 41, 45–47, 51–52, 69, 71, 75, 81, 85, 89–90, 94–95, 97, 99–100, 102–3, 106–8, 110, 116, 127–28, 134, 136–38, 144, 146, 148, 154–57, 162, 193, 195–97, 202, 204–5, 213,

216–18, 221, 235, 237, 273
big, 7, 41, 71
biggest, 52, 116
consulting, 75, 97, 202
nursing-home, 44, 107, 169, 194
real, 27, 102
well-managed, 28, 30

C

Capone, Al, 58–59
care plans, 124, 129, 131, 133, 165, 169, 200
Carington facility, 186–87
catch-22, 44
certification, 115, 187, 240
Chambery, Brook, 223–24
Chicago, Illinois, 58, 202, 225
Cicero, Illinois, 58
civil money penalties, 50, 57, 81, 107, 136, 138, 146, 153, 156, 160, 164, 170, 194, 219, 257
civil rights, 157–58, 164, 170
CMS (Centers for Medicare & Medicaid Services), 13, 25, 49, 61–62, 71–72, 74, 76–78, 81, 86–87, 97–98, 109–11, 124, 126, 136–37, 144–45, 148–49, 154, 156–57, 160–61, 172–75, 188, 192, 194, 206, 217–19, 226–27, 248, 257
CMS fines, 76–77
CNA (certified nursing assistant), 64, 104, 129–30, 132, 139, 143, 152, 174, 176, 186, 195, 205, 207–9, 211
commitment, 19, 144, 146, 186
Communist Manifesto, 39, 41–42
communist socialist state, 41
companionship, 237, 239–40
complaint

five-part, 102
survey, 76–77, 98, 144–46, 150–53, 175, 203
surveyor, 101–2
complaints, 46, 101, 106, 134–35, 141, 146–47, 160–61, 167, 174, 204–5, 218, 246
compliance, 64, 98, 120, 141, 144, 161, 168–69, 179, 195, 200, 209, 213
conditional license, 51, 77–78, 138, 154, 175–76, 205, 220
Congress, 9, 25, 34, 38, 53, 56–57, 62, 72, 93, 139–40, 215, 231, 242, 247, 252
Constitution, 43, 55, 57, 139–40, 233, 242
constitutional rights, 106, 141
consultant, 77–78, 110, 175, 187, 190, 193, 219–20, 225
Cooman, Kevin, 223
costs, 7–8, 10, 18, 23–25, 27–31, 52–53, 71, 73–74, 85, 88, 90, 94, 99, 110–13, 116, 118, 145, 151, 158, 174, 180, 187, 201, 203, 216, 221, 226, 232, 234, 238, 247–48, 255, 259, 261
  of attorneys, 73
  escalating, 52, 116
  fixed, 30–31, 235
  fraudulent, 62
  lower, 85, 187
  medication, 73, 180
  salary, 25
  semivariable, 29, 31
  variable, 31
coverage, 61, 74, 110, 191
CPR (cardiopulmonary resuscitation), 45, 77, 153–54, 176, 197, 207–12
Crystal (dietary manager), 176

D

damages, 136, 158, 191, 203
  punitive, 109, 141, 148, 157–58
defamation of owners, 157–58
deficiencies, 101, 104, 139, 141–42, 144, 147, 149, 151, 164–65, 226
denials, 59–60, 62, 73, 84, 155, 157
Department of Health and Human Services, 25, 71, 90, 106, 190, 247
Des Moines, Iowa, 78, 101, 157, 197, 219
Des Moines *Register*, 76, 78, 205, 220
DHS (Department of Human Services), 78, 161, 175, 219
DIA, director of, 79, 107–8, 195, 220
DIA (Department of Inspections and Appeals), 46, 55, 76, 78–79, 81, 120, 134, 144, 146, 152–54, 156–57, 159–61, 174–76, 193–95, 206, 211–13, 218–20, 246, 260–61
diagnoses, 17, 24, 52, 85, 94, 115, 129, 131, 163, 178
disabilities, 32, 48, 86, 94, 191, 235–36, 251
DRGs (diagnosis-related groupings), 7, 17, 19, 21, 52, 90, 115

E

economic incentives, 48, 109–10, 112, 118, 122, 125, 218, 234, 238, 248
economic problems, 39–40, 71
efficiency, 19, 22, 24–25, 89–90, 123, 126–28, 132
end-of-life sentence, 73–74
enforcement, 5, 9–11, 34, 55, 57, 71, 85, 87–90, 95, 106, 111, 115, 120, 216–17, 219, 221, 227
enforcement tactics, 59, 74, 81, 107, 110, 203, 217, 241
entitlements, 59, 71, 73, 231–35
entrapment, 45, 50, 81, 220
equality, 55, 139
evaluation, 116–17, 238
evidence, 56, 128, 133, 139–40, 154, 160, 174, 206–7, 211

F

failure, 49, 77, 126, 139, 165, 197–98, 201
fines, 46–47, 50, 76–78, 81–82, 88, 101, 103, 105, 108, 136, 138, 140–41, 145, 155, 157, 159–60, 173, 176, 197, 199–200, 204–5, 217–18, 220, 257, 259
floor incident, 76, 78, 220
Fox Valley facility, 133, 186
Fox v. Bowen, 61, 74, 110, 188–90, 196
fraud, 41, 57, 59–62, 74, 109, 163
fraud allegations, 62
freedom, 6, 37–39, 95, 171–72, 231
F-tags, 47, 103, 179, 226, 247

G

"gotcha," 107, 181, 193
government, 5, 7, 10, 17–19, 37–40, 44, 52–55, 57–60, 62–64, 70–71, 73–75, 85, 92–93, 95–96, 116, 122–23, 139, 190, 196, 203, 215, 217, 229–33, 235, 238, 246, 248–50, 252, 262
  corrupt, 70
government accountability, 43
government agencies, 59, 87
governmental fraud, 62

government appeals, 73
government buyers, 31
government claims, 60
government corruption, 70–72, 74, 163
government grants, 90, 159
government involvement, 59
government settlements, 62

H

HCFA (Health Care Financing Administration), 61
health care, 6–8, 14, 18–19, 21, 24–25, 29, 31, 34, 50, 52, 63–64, 71, 75, 83, 89, 109, 111, 114–15, 159, 171–72, 219, 225, 237, 245, 248, 252
  administration costs, 85
  business, 6, 32, 87
  industry, 212–13
  providers, 28–29, 45, 52, 83, 112, 115–16, 237
  system, 18, 83, 110, 112, 120, 236
health economics, 20, 23, 29
healthiest state, 107
health maintenance, 236–37
health preservation, 112, 236–37
HEW (Health Education and Welfare), 60, 73–74, 110, 219
HHS (Health and Human Services), 13, 137, 154, 156–57
Holman, Ed, 97
horizontal integration, 9, 30, 32
Hospital Corporation of America, 72

I

IDR (informal dispute review), 98, 103, 105, 143, 145, 156, 160–61, 172, 174
IDR hearings, 78, 148, 219
IDR process, 140, 142, 147, 151, 172
illness, 25, 72, 74, 87, 90, 216
  chronic, 236, 247
  spell of, 72, 102
immediate jeopardy (IJ), 77, 98, 141–42, 154, 165–66, 171–72, 176, 206, 211, 255, 257
inaccuracies, factual, 152
incentives, 18–19, 25, 33–34, 109, 113, 117, 123, 216, 219, 234
  moral, 91, 109, 112, 118, 234
incontinence, 142, 148
incontinence care, 142, 148, 201
innovation, 6, 50, 197, 250
insanity, 101–2, 107
interventions, 72, 78, 81, 86, 116–17, 129, 131, 142, 177–78, 219
investigation, 82, 102, 138, 150, 152, 154, 160–61, 165–66, 168, 172, 207, 209, 211–12
Iowa Department of Inspections and Appeals, 76, 199, 212, 215, 260
irreparable harm, 137

J

Jimmo v. Sibelius, 61, 74, 137, 189, 191, 196
judicial power, 56, 140
judicial review, 56, 139

K

Kithil (judge), 92–93
Klaassen, Joni, 134–35

L

labor, 20, 30–31, 42, 119, 261
labor component, 23–24
labor costs, 28–29, 31, 73, 131
labor efficiency, 30–31
Lexington facility, 163, 165–73
life sentence, 73–74
Little Rock, Arkansas, 95, 97, 99, 215

M

Marx, Karl, 39, 41
maximum standards, 123–24
MDS (minimum data set), 110, 165, 169, 225–26
Medicaid, 60, 62, 64, 73–75, 84–85, 87, 99, 109–11, 119, 137, 153, 168, 171, 179–80, 190–91, 215–16, 219, 235, 248
Medicare, 28, 38, 59–60, 62, 72–73, 75, 79, 84, 87, 99, 110–11, 137, 141, 165, 168, 171, 179–80, 188–91, 195, 219–20, 235, 248
Medicare benefits, 48, 59–60, 64, 86, 93, 155, 185, 190, 196, 215
Medicare billings, 188
Medicare cases, 186, 189
Medicare claims, 60–62, 73, 192
  denied, 62
  incidence of, 73
  unfiled, 62
Medicare coverage, 74, 191–92
Medicare module, 202–3
Medicare money, 32, 78, 237
Medicare overpayment, 59
Medicare Part A, 60–61
Medicare patients, 179, 187
Medicare program, 59, 71, 79, 190, 192, 220, 256

medications
  inappropriate, 117, 119
  psychotropic, 165–66
Michelle (LPN), 207–10
minimum standards, 10, 121–24, 152, 199, 247
mom-and-pops, 23, 30, 32, 71, 162
monopsony, 7, 9, 11, 17, 19–21, 25, 30, 45, 50, 63, 70, 163, 221, 230, 235, 246–48, 252–54, 258–59, 261
Monopsony Game, 8, 17, 34, 82, 115, 229
Muscatine, Iowa, 63, 76, 95, 100, 102, 137, 144, 149, 151–52, 174, 176, 193–96, 202, 204, 212, 215–16, 226, 257
Muscatine facility, 76, 79, 100, 107, 109, 152, 220, 226, 258

N

noncompliant facility, 78–79, 219
nonpayment, 74
numerical deficit, 178

O

Obama Care, 6, 11, 17–18, 41, 60, 62, 73, 85, 88, 93, 205
one-buyer market, 17, 20, 28, 31, 33
  government-owned, 17
on-site surveyors, 82, 160
operating losses, 79, 157, 162, 193, 220
Oz, 70

P

patient-abuse policies, 175
patient care, 45, 106, 146, 193, 223
patients, 5, 14, 17, 27, 29, 33–34,

46–48, 50, 55, 59–61, 63–64, 72–79, 81, 83, 85, 93, 99, 103–5, 108–10, 118–20, 123–24, 128–29, 131–33, 136, 138–39, 141, 143, 146–47, 149–50, 152–61, 173–75, 177–78, 180, 185–87, 189–90, 194–97, 203–6, 208–11, 213, 216–19, 221, 226–27, 239–41, 246, 250–51, 255, 259, 261
- abused, 154, 211
- adoption of a, 239
- ambulatory, 186
- behavior problem, 147
- behavior-problem, 103
- care, 176
- complex care, 153
- critical-care, 180
- delusional, 78, 220
- depressed, 227
- discharge, 119, 161
- elderly, 72–73
- expired, 206
- functional, 185
- goal, 86
- heavy-care, 32
- incontinent, 101
- longer-term care, 33
- mistreating, 204
- noncompliant, 46, 106, 161
- private-pay, 30
- restored, 203
- safety, 83
- troubled geriatric-psychiatric, 153

penalties, 50, 82, 88, 122, 140–41, 145, 155, 160–61, 247
plaintiffs, 134, 136–38, 155–56, 158, 192
productivity, 18, 22, 25, 29–31, 126–27
productivity levels, 21, 25

profit margins, 17–18, 27
profits, 18–20, 24–26, 29, 33–34, 41, 45, 126, 230, 232, 235
programming, 117–19, 187, 237
  restorative, 73, 117–18, 165, 261
proof, 5, 36, 64, 106, 154, 207, 219
Provider Bill of Rights, 159, 196, 218
provider number, 97, 144–45, 157
provider rights, 51, 159–60
providers, 6–7, 9, 14, 17–18, 25, 28–29, 32, 45, 49–52, 55, 59–62, 73–76, 81, 87, 89, 101–3, 106–7, 109–11, 113, 116, 121–23, 125, 135–36, 139, 141, 145, 151, 155–61, 190–92, 203, 215, 218, 221, 239, 245–47, 255
- cost-efficient, 29
- effective, 149
- efficient, 18
- independent, 194
- insensitive, 240
- intimidated, 109
- nursing-facility, 122
- punished, 136

punishment, 55, 76, 102, 136, 144, 154, 156, 175, 211, 214, 220
punitive actions, 79, 81, 205, 220
punitive relief, 157–58

Q

QOC (quality of care), 238
QOL (quality of life), 238–39, 245
quality incentive payment, 48, 118, 133, 186
QUIP (quality incentive payment), 118, 120, 186

R

Reagan, Ronald Wilson
  (president), 39–41
Reck, Rob, 77, 135, 143, 174, 204–5
record review, 142
recovery, 17, 59–60, 165, 245
reimbursement, 29, 103, 110, 122,
  226, 247
relief, 137, 144, 156, 158
  injunctive, 134–36
renovations, 64, 80, 100
Republican, 41, 113
resolution, 106, 161, 191
restoration, 64, 102, 238, 245
restorative care, 63–64, 193–94
restorative-care facilities, 212
restorative model, 99, 108, 180,
  194, 225–26, 238
restorative services, 18, 63, 110,
  112–13, 165, 168, 238, 240
retaliation, 51, 76, 78–79, 81,
  107–8, 115, 141, 144, 151,
  154, 157–58, 174, 194–96,
  220, 261
Rhoads, George, 13, 184
Rhoads, Kip, 13–14, 76, 78–79, 97,
  104, 148–49, 174, 180, 193,
  202–3, 220
Rhoads, Sharon, 163, 211, 237
RICO Act (Racketeer Influenced
  and Corrupt Organizations
  Act), 58
rigor mortis, 154, 197, 207–11
Roberts, Rod, 64, 76, 107–8, 120,
  144, 176, 246
RUGs (resource-utilization
  groups), 7, 18, 52, 90, 110,
  116, 183

S

severity, 46, 72, 78, 141–42, 145,
  151, 160, 165
  level of, 98, 151
severity codes, 82, 101, 103, 138, 155
Smith, Adam, 19, 22–23
special-focus designation, 76, 154, 157
spiritual rehab, 118–19
stars of quality, 117, 123–24, 186
state fines, 76–77, 154, 173
substandard care, 10, 105, 143,
  151, 166, 170, 175, 205, 217
surveys, extended, 77, 172–73

T

T., Richard, 77, 153–54, 176, 207–8
Teresa (LPN), 207–10
Thatcher, Margaret, 39–40
Transmittal 262, 14, 61, 188–90

V

violations, 10, 45, 56, 76–78, 98,
  101, 104–6, 123, 138, 140,
  144–45, 153, 157, 161, 163,
  165–66, 168–70, 172, 176,
  190, 196, 201, 204–5, 246–47
  level, 97, 103–4, 151

W

White, Dorotha C., 13, 166,
  170–72
Wills, Marty, 149, 174
Woodland Terrace, 198–201

Other Books Written by Jerry L. Rhoads

Jerry Rhoads, the author, has written magazine articles, books, manuscripts, and training materials for his accounting and consulting business for thirty-seven years. Many have been published by industry magazines and periodicals. Others are published by his company Caregiver Management Systems for training his clients. Now the books are being presented to publishers for review and acceptance.

The Basic Accounting and Budgeting for Long Term Care Facilities (1981), published by CBI Publishing Company Inc., Boston, Massachusetts, underwritten by the American Health Care Association, and published by CBI Publishing as a part of Mr. Rhoads's authorship of the current Prospective Payment System.

Basic Accounting and Budgeting for Long Term Care Facilities, Second Edition (1978), published by American Health Care Association

Never Too Old to Live (2012), published by Xlibris
The Boomers Are Coming (2012), published by Xlibris
Remedy Eldercide Restore Elder Pride (2009), published by iUniverse
Restore Elder Pride (2013, second edition), published by iUniverse
American Enterprise Manifesto (2013), published by Xlibris
America in the Red Zone (2013), published by iUniverse

Published by Caregiver Management Systems

How to Win the Monopsony Game (2002–2008)
Medicare Expert Handbook (2004–2007)
Become a Flagship in Your Market, an e-book on www.ecaregiver.com, October 2008
Mechanics of Quality and Profit for Skilled Nursing Facilities (2002)

The Monopsony Game, a board game created by Jerry Roads, can be ordered through the website *jrhoads@allamericancare.com*.

www.ingramcontent.com/pod-product-compliance
Lightning Source LLC
Chambersburg PA
CBHW020735180526
45163CB00001B/249